Living with the AIDS Virus

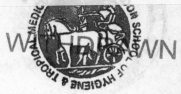

Living with the AIDS Virus

The Epidemic and the Response in India

Editors

Samiran Panda
Anindya Chatterjee
Abu S. Abdul-Quader

SAGE Publications
New Delhi • Thousand Oaks • London

Copyright © Samiran Panda, 2002

First published in 2002 by

Sage Publications India Pvt Ltd
M–32 Market, Greater Kailash I
New Delhi 110 048

Sage Publications Inc.
2455 Teller Road
Thousand Oaks, California 91320

Sage Publications Ltd
6 Bonhill Street
London EC2A 4PU

Published by Tejeshwar Singh for Sage Publications India Pvt Ltd, Typeset by C&M Digitals (P) Ltd., Chennai in 10/12 New Baskerville and printed at Chaman Enterprises, Delhi.

Library of Congress Cataloging-in-Publication Data

Living with the AIDS virus : the epidemic and the response in India / editors, Samiran Panda, Anindya Chatterjee, and Abu S. Abdul-Quader.
    p.cm.
    Includes bibliographical references and index.
    1. AIDS (Disease)—India. I. Panda, Samiran, 1960- II. Chatterjee, Anindya, 1961- III. Abdul-Quader, Abu S., 1950–

RA643.86.I42 L48   362.1'969792'0954—dc21   2002   2002026886

ISBN: 0-7619-9622-2 (US-Hb)   81-7829-168-1 (India-Hb)
       0-7619-9623-0 (US-Pb)   81-7829-169-X (India-Pb)

Sage Production Team: Dipika Nath, K.E. Priyamvada, Sushanta Gayen and Santosh Rawat

To

People Living with HIV/AIDS and their Friends
(PLWHAF)

Contents

Foreword

All over the world, the spread of HIV/AIDS has initially generated fear which, in turn, has led to blaming. Blaming reinforces negative sociocultural stereotypes and leads to further marginalisation of those most at risk. However, a vital lesson from the global tragedy on HIV/AIDS shows that rather than being targets of blame, fear and alienating rhetoric, the secrets of success in HIV/AIDS prevention lie in having a mindset that sees groups at risk as teachers and colleagues. Clearly, teachers need tools, whether educative skills with which to strengthen community responses and interventions, or contextual, such as workable legislative structures, community education and awareness, health services and economic and social enfranchisement. No country has succeeded in fighting HIV/AIDS by denial, judgementalism or blaming. Such responses as these drive epidemics underground and amplify the fatal silence in which the virus flourishes.

Through such a perspective, HIV/AIDS is seen irreducibly as a developmental phenomenon. The current book, which is a detailed examination of the national response to HIV/AIDS in India, reveals some remarkable success stories and interventions whilst also showing that the national response to HIV/AIDS remains a work in progress.

India has some world-class models of interventions for prevention which reveal the importance of using those communities being targeted as part of the solution, not as the problem. The book highlights the challenge of partnerships that intersect many agendas while forging new ones. It also highlights the complexity of the epidemic in India. Challenges to rational and sustained intervention include the diversity of cultural norms and the centrality of many of them, as well as the challenges of stigma, gender inequality, migration, poverty, the prevalence of sexually transmitted diseases, commercial sex and its wilful invisibility, difficulties in discussing sex with youth, and legislative restrictions, to name but a few.

Many new initiatives have been undertaken since the manuscript was written. These include the expansion of sero-surveillance for HIV to 320 sites; the development of the Family Health Awareness Campaigns which, to date, have reached over 70 million people; the piloting and subsequent plans for expansion of mother-to-child transmission prevention; and the development of a coherent political response at national and state levels. Even more recently, a national AIDS policy has been published for the first time in India. Recent months have also seen the publication of results from the extraordinary behavioural sentinel surveillance undertaken nationally.

While shedding new light on the penetration of HIV education and intervention efforts, the recent behavioural sentinel surveillance data also reveal new challenges. For example, while the majority of the population in India has heard of HIV/AIDS, in many states the minority of the population can only draw a link between sexually transmitted infections and HIV.

The book is at its best in revealing such complexities and such challenges. It draws lessons from the Indian experiences that are in many ways global lessons. They include, in addition to those already suggested, basic responses that are easy to write but extremely difficult at times to implement:

- Overcoming ignorance and the invisibility of the present epidemic through creative and relevant educational efforts that assist in personalising HIV/AIDS and the responsibilities of individuals;
- Giving recognition to areas of risk that society would often prefer to ignore, such as commercial sex work, men having sex with men, injecting drug use, and the oft-cited double standards in Indian sexuality that put women particularly at risk;
- The need for adequate and dedicated staff appropriately trained in the complexities of HIV counselling and clinical management;
- The critical importance of validating assumptions upon which a comprehensive national sero-surveillance is translated into prevalence estimates for both HIV/AIDS and for AIDS mortality;

- The importance of educating both health staff and mainstream populations in the challenges of HIV and responsibilities of prevention;
- The need to lift the deathly veil of denial at the social and legislative and political levels;
- Using an environmental/contextual focus in the design and implementation of targeted interventions;
- The critical importance of enabling access to voluntary counselling and testing—people must know their vulnerability if they are to be motivated to act in order to reduce it;
- Strengthening options for care through existing health services;
- The importance of establishing partnerships that work up from the realities of community experience, not down from the realities of a centrist perspective;
- The vital need to maintain adherence to quality in interventions of all types;
- The need to bridge the resource gap between what is available and what is required whilst at the same time enhancing absorption capacity (another very good reason for community empowerment as a central focus of future intervention efforts).

These Indian and global lessons also reveal that in the second most HIV/AIDS infected country on earth, the Indian national response must learn from the experiences of other countries if that response is to meaningfully connect with and reverse current epidemic trends in the country. HIV/AIDS is a global phenomenon, not merely a national one. Lessons of success and failure can and must be imported as well as exported from state to state and from nation to nation. This excellent book helps to show those areas in which such necessary exchange may yield greater benefit. The authors and editors should be congratulated for assisting all those working in HIV/AIDS prevention, care and support in India in learning how we can use vital lessons from the recent tragic history of this phenomenon in India.

Dr David Miller
Country Programme Advisor
UNAIDS (India)

Preface

As of March 2001, India had 20,304 reported cases of acquired immunodeficiency syndrome (AIDS) and many more human immunodeficiency virus (HIV) infections. Given the size of the country, high population density, and interstate movement of people, the control of the spread of the virus becomes more critical and urgent in India. In Africa, HIV is spread mostly through heterosexual transmission. In India, HIV appears to be spreading through various modes of transmission, including risk behaviours such as injection drug use. Because of the presence of multiple risk behaviours and factors, HIV is spreading widely and fast.

Since the beginning of the epidemic in India, in 1986, a variety of interventions have been implemented targeting different population groups and there has been a wide spectrum of responses at the local as well as international levels. Various government and non-governmental organisations (NGOs) have designed, developed and implemented HIV prevention interventions in different parts of the country. Some of these have been indigenous, and others have been based on experiences from other parts of the world. Some of these interventions have made significant impact in terms of reaching the populations at risk and bringing changes in behaviours. Given the present state of the epidemic as well as the estimated number of infections, it is not only important to document the current prevention efforts in the country, but also to examine their efficacy, implications and the necessary future directions.

This book focuses on the HIV/AIDS situation in India as it relates to the epidemiology of, and responses to, the epidemic, specifically in the programmes for prevention and care currently being implemented in the country. It has been written by experts working in the field of HIV/AIDS in India and the subcontinent.

Chapter 1 provides an overview of the HIV/AIDS epidemic in India. It highlights the epidemiology of HIV/AIDS in the country, with particular reference to the HIV/AIDS situation in severely affected states and union territories. For each state and union territory discussed, references will be made to the HIV/AIDS situation as it relates to different risk behaviours.

Chapter 2 deals with the government response to HIV/AIDS in India. Given the federal structure of the government, and that health is under the jurisdiction of state authority, the chapter describes government responses both at the central and the state levels. It critically reviews government responses in each of the areas of prevention, intervention (including condom promotion and distribution), blood safety, programme management, care, and legal and ethical issues, as well as looks at some of the successes and some of the gaps in the responses.

Chapter 3 focuses specifically on NGO responses to HIV/AIDS in India. Since the beginning of the epidemic, NGOs worldwide have taken a leading role in promoting safe behaviours and implementing community-based interventions. This is being done very successfully in Africa and has been happening in India as well. This chapter critically examines the roles the NGOs have played in terms of implementing interventions and promoting safer behaviours, and how these NGO responses help in the fight against HIV/AIDS.

Chapter 4 deals with the sociocultural environment in which the HIV epidemic is breeding now in India and highlights the importance of environmental intervention that should be given due importance while attempting behaviour modification.

There are a number of HIV/AIDS prevention interventions currently being implemented in various parts of the country and it is important to document not only the positive aspects of these interventions but also the problems encountered in implementing the programmes, especially the responses at the community level. Chapters 5 to 8 deal with community responses to HIV/AIDS and specific HIV/AIDS interventions targeting injecting drug users (IDUs), sex workers (SWs) and men who have sex with men (MSM). These examples serve as lessons learned from the field and can then be replicated in other parts of the country.

Chapter 9 deals with the legal issues related to HIV/AIDS in India. As the epidemic gradually attains a stage of advancement in the country, many intricate concerns come to the fore. The law is yet to face the whole array of these issues, and a more comprehensive response is likely to take shape in the future. This chapter initiates the reader towards this understanding.

Chapter 10 identifies the strengths as well as weaknesses of the interventions and also highlights the very important aspect of the socio-economic impact of HIV/AIDS, which has so far remained neglected in almost all the intervention programmes in India. If the people responsible for developing and implementing interventions to prevent the spread of HIV/AIDS—policymakers at local, national and international levels, and the national and international funding agencies working in India and the subregion of the continent—find this book useful, the efforts that have gone into bringing out this publication will be worth spent.

Samiran Panda
Anindya Chatterjee
Abu S. Abdul-Quader

Acknowledgements

As is inevitable with a publication of this nature, we are indebted to many scholars, policymakers and interventionists working in India and the subcontinent for helping us to decide on what should appear as chapters in this book. Preparing an exhaustive list of all of them is difficult. However, we would be failing in our duty if we do not mention that Mr Tejeshwar Singh and Ms Deepa Pahari of Sage India Pvt Ltd sowed the seed of this book on a dusty afternoon during the 'Calcutta Book Fair–1995' when two of us (SP and AC) met them.

India by then had already entered the second decade of an HIV epidemic and there were many useful experiences of public health importance that were worth documenting. However there was no book that served this end, and there still isn't one. The credit goes to Ms Omita Goyal of Sage who subsequently took the onus on herself to water the seed sown at the Calcutta Book Fair. She was tireless in writing us letters, sending e-mails and ensuring the progress of this project. Since then much water has flown down the river Ganges and Calcutta has changed its name to Kolkata. Finally, the team of Sage comprising Ms Dipika Nath, Ms K.E. Priyamvada and Mr Amarjyoti Dutta with their unwavering determination, brought the project to its completion. Without them it would just not have been possible to walk those extra miles.

We acknowledge the positive gesture of Dr David Miller, the country Programme Advisor of UNAIDS, India, who kindly agreed to write the foreword for the book in spite of his busy schedule. Mr Subodh Karmakar of the National Institute of Cholera and Enteric Diseases (ICMR) and Mr Krishanu Deb Barman of the Society for Applied Studies, Kolkata extended their valuable secretarial assistance during the preparation of the manuscript.

Our sincere appreciation also goes to all the contributors who have given their time and expertise in writing and modifying the chapters based on the peer-reviewer's comments.

Finally, we are grateful to many physicians, government employees, people living with HIV/AIDS, and NGOs from all over the country who knew about the making of this book and constantly kept us inspired by asking when they could actually lay their hands on the finished product.

1

The HIV/AIDS Epidemic in India: An Overview

Samiran Panda

Introduction

The estimated global total of adults and children afflicted by HIV/AIDS[1] was 34.3 million in 1999, approximately 16 per cent of which (5.6 million) was from South and South-East Asia—the region with half of the world's population (UNAIDS 2000). Given the tremendous cultural, geographic and economic diversity of Asian countries, patterns of HIV transmission vary among the different nations. In most countries in Asia, the majority of HIV transmission among adults is through heterosexual intercourse and the sharing of injecting equipment among injecting drug users (IDUs). However, a substantial amount of transmission is also caused by male-to-male sex and by transfusion of HIV-infected blood/blood products (Mastro et al. 1998).

HIV was first detected in India in 1986, five years after the detection of AIDS in the United States of America. Although it was known by then from the experiences of other countries that the virus would not spare any caste, creed, colour or race, India, like many other countries, went through a phase of denial before accepting it as a major public health problem. The heterogeneous spread of HIV within the country especially made the less affected states and union territories think that it was not a real issue for them—a trend that exists till today in a different form. Some of the relatively less affected states expected that awareness campaigns would mount an effective barrier against the spread of HIV, although there is abundant evidence that not just awareness but also making other means of behaviour change available would be required to slow down the further spread of the virus. Taking cognisance of 'vulnerability' and developing interventions around it came into practice much later, and that too happened on a limited scale.

The epidemiological evidence of the spread of HIV in the country in the early 1990s gave rise to national-level public health efforts for its containment with support from WHO and World Bank. Since then a decade has passed. It is now evident that, in order to be effective, the HIV/AIDS control programme needs to be related to larger health issues, including health service delivery performance in different states. It is also becoming obvious that any HIV/AIDS intervention plan in India needs to take into account the country-specific contexts as well as constraints because, otherwise, the development of sustainable and efficient intervention programmes will not be possible. Poverty, which makes the risk of AIDS an important matter for the poor; the powerlessness of women, which makes negotiation of safer sex an impractical proposition; and inadequate supplies of clean syringes and needles, which make safer injecting behaviour impossible are some of the concerns in this regard (Priya 1994). The creation of an enabling environment for safer behaviour is thus critically important in India.

HIV/AIDS in India: The Current Scenario and Behaviour Surveillance Survey (BSS)

As of March 2001, India has reported a cumulative total of 20,304 cases of AIDS; 15,563 males and 4,741 females (NACO 2000–2001) while the estimated number of HIV infections is 3.9 million. Although the spread of HIV infection in the country has mostly been driven by heterosexual transmission, more opportunities for men to access health care facilities could probably explain this difference in the reported number of AIDS cases across gender. It should also be noted that younger women married to older men in different states of India have contracted HIV infection from their husbands (many of whom are in an advanced stage of HIV disease during marriage) and would reach the stage of AIDS later than their husbands as it is known from the natural history of HIV disease that a younger age of acquiring the infection is inversely related to the progression to AIDS. In 83 per cent of the reported cases of AIDS, HIV infection has been acquired through the sexual route, 4 per cent through sharing of injection equipment during drug use and another 4 per cent through contaminated blood/blood product transfusion. Perinatal transmission accounts for 2 per cent of the total cases of AIDS. As many children in different states including the ones worst hit by HIV epidemic in the country die of opportunistic infections without attending any hospital, it is not difficult to assume that many cases of paediatric AIDS are yet to be reflected in reports. In 7 per cent of the reported AIDS cases, the history of the route of transmission is not available. The age-wise distribution of AIDS cases reported from all over the country reveals that 50 per cent of the total male (6,022/15,563) and female AIDS cases (1,692/4,741) falls within the age range of 15–29 years which has a great implication for the overall socio-economic development of the country.

The recent countrywide 'Behaviour Surveillance Survey' (BSS) conducted among the general population as opposed to surveys earlier conducted in groups observing high-risk behaviour is the biggest of its kind in the world. It was conducted during April–September 2001 when a total of 84,478 respondents were interviewed in which males and females participated in equal proportion; urban and rural representation was also equal in this survey (NACO 2001). Seventy-six per cent of the respondents in this survey had ever heard of HIV/AIDS (82.4 per cent males and 70 per cent females); low awareness was recorded among rural women in Bihar, Gujarat, Uttar Pradesh, Madhya Pradesh and West Bengal. This finding is particularly important in view of the fact that the epidemic is now making inroads into rural areas as well as in women representing the general female population in India. Overall 8.7 per cent of the respondents in the BSS reported that they knew or heard of somebody suffering from HIV/AIDS; the highest proportion was in Manipur (37 per cent) and Andhra Pradesh (36.7 per cent). Moreover, nearly one in 10 respondents in the country knew or heard of someone who died of AIDS. Such experiences were most commonly reported from Manipur (37 per cent), Andhra Pradesh (31 per cent) and Maharashtra (21 per cent). All these responses indicate that the HIV epidemic has now become a palpable reality to many in the country and is sure to impact on resource utilisation and deprivation at the levels of institutions, communities as well as on the household and family. It is also important to note that condom use with non-regular sex partners, particularly consistent condom use with all non-regular partners in the last 12 months, was reported to be very low in many states like Assam, Bihar, Karnataka, Manipur, Madhya Pradesh and Uttar Pradesh.

HIV Surveillance

A countrywide surveillance for HIV was initiated in India in 1985 (ICMR 1988). Its focus was on people observing high-risk sexual and/or drug use behaviour. In 1986, HIV was detected in a group of female sex workers (SWs) from Chennai—previously called Madras (John et al. 1987). Subsequently, the virus was detected in female SWs of Mumbai (previously called Bombay), a coastal metropolitan city in western India. The prevalence of HIV in Mumbai SWs gradually went up, from 0 per cent in 1987 to 20 per cent within a period of three years (WHO 1993).

A rapid spread of HIV among IDUs was observed in the three north-eastern states of India bordering Myanmar (Manipur, Mizoram and Nagaland) in the late 1980s. Within six months of the entry of HIV in Manipur, 50 per cent of the local injectors of heroin (purest variety, locally known as 'white sugar' or 'number 4') were infected with the virus. It may be noted that from 1986 through September 1989, no HIV was detected by sero-surveillance conducted among IDUs in Manipur (Sarkar et al. 1993). The exact time of the entry of HIV is thus known for Manipur, and studying the future course of the epidemic and responses to it in this state could lend many important lessons to practitioners of public health.

The north-eastern state of Mizoram recorded a 10 per cent HIV prevalence among local injectors in 1991. IDUs in Mizoram, due to the non-availability of injectable heroin, following stringent customs activity in the late 1980s, started injecting dextropropoxyphene after dissolving the synthetic powder emptied from the capsules of spasmoproxyvon obtained from peddlers or procured over the counter. Subsequent surveillance data from the State AIDS Control Society of Mizoram showed a stable HIV prevalence in IDUs, ranging from 5 to 10 per cent, over the next eight years. However, a rise in heterosexual transmission of HIV gradually took over in Mizoram during this time. A change in the drug injecting pattern was seen in Manipur in the early 2000, similar to the trend in Mizoram in the late 1980s, when users switched to injecting dextropropoxyphene, as white sugar became non-available and costly.

The general notion that prevailed was that injection drug use-related HIV would pose a problem for north-east India due to its geographical proximity to Myanmar, a country with large illegal poppy plant cultivation (opium, extracted from poppy pod, is used to prepare morphine, which is in turn converted to heroin through chemical treatment). However, this notion was subsequently proved wrong. The spread of injection drug use started to be observed in major metropolitan cities such as Kolkata (previously known as Calcutta), Delhi and Chennai during the mid- and late-1990s, and HIV also made inroads in IDUs in these places (Dorabjee et al. 1996, Kumar et al. 1997, Panda et al. 1997). In Kolkata and Delhi, the drug of choice for injecting was buprenorphine (synthetic opioid painkiller) but in Chennai, injection of both buprenorphine and brown sugar (adulterated heroin, which is generally smoked and needs to be heated with vitamin C tablets or lemon juice for dissolving before injecting) was recorded. A large number of brown sugar smokers in these cities switched to injecting buprenorphine, as buprenorphine was comparatively cheaper and capable of combating the withdrawal symptoms suffered by brown sugar smokers during the heroin drought (Panda et al. 1997) due to police seizures. In some cases, brown sugar smokers admitted in detoxification centres came to know about the use of buprenorphine injection from the physicians treating them with the medicine and, after being discharged from the centres, switched to injecting buprenorphine during relapse.

Similar to the phenomenon of the diffusion of HIV in IDUs in several cities in India, the spread of HIV through the heterosexual route also did not remain restricted to the states of Tamil Nadu and Maharashtra, where it was first detected. Sexually transmitted disease (STD) clinics in Vasco da Gama, the largest town in the

Table 1.1

Data on cumulative numbers* of reported HIV and AIDS cases

Year	HIV Seropositivity Rate (per 1000)	Cumulative Number of AIDS Cases
1986	2.5	6
1988	3.5	14
1990	5.2	60
1992	10.2	290
1994	13.4	1,017
1996	16.8	3,161
1998	22.7	5,204

Source: Country Scenario, Update 1991 NACP, 1997–2000 NACO reports.
*As of March 2000, 11,251 AIDS cases had been reported to NACO. This figure is considered to be only a fraction of the true picture due to under-reporting accruing from the limitations of the existing surveillance system (NACO 1999–2000).

state of Goa, recorded a staggering growth of HIV prevalence, from 1 per cent in 1987 to 27 per cent in 1993 (NACO 1995).

A rise in HIV seropositivity was found to be a consistent phenomenon in almost all states, irrespective of the time of first detection in particular states. No HIV case was reported in Orissa till the end of 1992, but the estimated seropositivity rate there, as of November 1995, was 2.44/1000 (ibid.). The cumulative number of reported HIV and AIDS cases for the country thus gradually reached a high figure (Table 1.1) with a sudden jump observed in 1995 (2,108 cases of AIDS being reported in 1995, compared to 1,017 cases in 1994). While the number of AIDS cases in 1995 reflected on the incidence[2] rate of HIV in the late 1980s (50 per cent of HIV-infected people, who do not receive anti-retroviral therapy, reach the stage of AIDS by eight years), it is acknowledged by the government that the actual number of AIDS cases in the community would be much higher (NACO 1999–2000).

HIV Types and Subtypes in India

All the states in India now have a reported presence of HIV—the predominant type being HIV-1. HIV-2 also has a wide geographical distribution in the country but has infected a fewer number of people. HIV-2 is apparently less transmissible and causes AIDS more slowly as compared to HIV-1.

The first evidence of HIV-2 came in 1991 from the northern part of India, where paid blood donors and STD clinic attendees were found to be infected with it (Chattopadhya et al. 1991). Subsequently, HIV-2 was detected in Bihar (Saran and Gupta 1995), Maharashtra (Kulkarni et al. 1992), Goa (Rubsamen-Waigmann et al. 1992), Chennai (Solomon and Ganapathy 1992) and Vellore (Babu et al. 1993), the infection being acquired in all these places through heterosexual contact. The only report documenting HIV-2 in injecting drug users came from Manipur. Finding HIV-2 in injectors is unusual as this type of HIV has been found to spread mostly through the heterosexual route. Five of the 76 IDUs (7 per cent) in this study from Manipur were dually infected with HIV-1 and HIV-2 in 1994; none was exclusively infected with HIV-2 (Singh et al. 1995). Sixty-one per cent (46 out of 76) of the IDUs in the same study had only HIV-1. As HIV-1 was the predominant type of human immunodeficiency virus in Manipur and HIV-2 was not reported from the neighbouring countries of Thailand and Myanmar, it was presumed that HIV-2 in Manipur might have spread through the sexual exposure of travellers who returned to Manipur from other areas of India. Young men in Manipur frequently leave the state temporarily, either for education or employment, or to reduce their access to heroin. It is also possible that these men acquire HIV-2 sexually while in other parts of India and transport it back to Manipur. Evidence of the presence of HIV-2 in India made stronger the case for adopting a test system in the country that could detect antibodies for both HIV-1 and HIV-2.

Subtype distribution of HIV-1 within the country, with its implications for vaccine development, has been a matter of immense interest among molecular biologists. Subtype C of HIV-1 accounts for the largest proportion of infections in India; the next common being subtype B, Thai-B and Thai-A, in descending order (Mastro et al. 1998).

Changed Surveillance Strategy

Sentinel surveillance was adopted in India during 1993–94 to circumvent the inherent limitations of the cumulative sero-surveillance data. HIV sentinel surveillance aims at unlinked anonymous testing of a predetermined number of blood samples (250 for population groups observing high-risk behaviour and

400 for low-risk populations) collected from selected sites (clinics) within a limited period of time (four to six weeks), at regular intervals. This helps in quick appraisal of changes in HIV prevalence in different population groups as well as the entry of the virus in new populations. It also has the potential for indirect examination of the adequacy of existing interventions. Activities for sentinel surveillance include testing STD clinic attendees and IDUs for HIV in an unlinked anonymous way as representative of people observing moderate- and high-risk behaviour respectively. Antenatal clinic (ANC) attendees, on the other hand, are tested as representative of the general female population. Each state conducts one round of sentinel surveillance every year.

A decline in the performance of sentinel surveillance by the states was observed in 1996, which improved in 1997–98 (NACO 1996). The distribution of sentinel surveillance sites all over the country is shown in Table 1.2.

The latest sentinel surveillance report reveals that HIV has made inroads in the general population through heterosexual

Table 1.2
HIV sentinel sites in India*

Total States/Union Territories	32
States/Union Territories—with Sites	32
States/Union Territories—without Sites	Nil
Number of sentinel sites	
Sites till 1996–97	55
Additional Sites—1997–98	125
Total Sites	180
Number of sites as per sentinel groups	
STD	79
ANC	71
ANC-R**	18
IDU	07
Blood Donors	01
Truckers	02
TB patients	02

Source: Country Scenario 1997–98, National AIDS Control Organisation,
Ministry of Health and Family Welfare, Government of India.
*In 2000 a total of 237 select sites were used from all over the country. Of this 109 were STD clinics, 110 clinics for pregnant women, 11 sites for IDUs and only two for MSM.
**Antenatal clinic a rural area.

transmission, and the epidemic has progressed in rural areas as well. Based on the analysis of sentinel surveillance data from 2000, the states and union territories in India have been broadly classified into three groups:

- Group I includes states such as Maharashtra, Tamil Nadu, Karnataka, Andhra Pradesh, Manipur and Nagaland, where HIV prevalence[3] is above 5 per cent in population groups observing high-risk behaviour (for example, sex workers and/or IDUs) and 1 per cent or more in antenatal women (representing the general female population).
- Group II includes states/union territories such as Gujarat, Goa, West Bengal, Delhi, Kerala, Mizoram and Pondicherry, where HIV prevalence has crossed 5 per cent among people observing high-risk behaviour but the infection is below 1 per cent in antenatal women.
- Group III includes the remaining states, where the HIV prevalence in any of the population groups observing high-risk behaviour is still less then 5 per cent and less than 1 per cent of antenatal women are infected with HIV.

The estimated numbers of HIV-infected people in the country calculated on the basis of sentinel surveillance data are 3.5 million, 3.7 million and 3.9 million for 1998, 1999 and 2000 respectively. However, the estimates mainly focused on people belonging to the 15–49 years age group and did not take into account the reported cases of AIDS. The latest estimate of 3.97 million HIV-infected people for 2001 has been pointed out as a probable slowing down of the epidemic by the government.

HIV Disease and AIDS in the Country

A cohort of infected people, followed up prospectively for a few years from the onset of infection, is essential for studying the natural history of any chronic, infectious disease, particularly for a disease such as AIDS, where the incubation period for clinical illnesses following infection varies for most of the people from five to eight years (without anti-HIV medicines). Lack of adequate funds, shifts in priorities of funding agencies for HIV research in developing countries and lack of investigation facilities, especially for cell mediated immunity studies in places worst hit by HIV, have been responsible for the dearth of information from India in this regard.

Data on opportunistic infections as well as other manifestation associated with HIV in the country has mostly been generated through case reports, cross-sectional studies and autopsy findings. The common symptomatic presentation of HIV in India includes persistent generalised lymphadenopathy (PGL), herpes zoster (reactivation of the dormant chicken pox virus), oral thrush (fungal infection of the mouth), and long-continued diarrhoea where causative organisms remain unknown in many situations (Lanjewar, Rodrigues et al. 1996), pulmonary and extrapulmonary tuberculosis, prolonged fever and cachexia (Kaur et al. 1992, Panda, Kamei et al. 1994, Sen et al. 1993). Tuberculosis topped the list of opportunistic infections associated with the reported cases of AIDS in India (NACO 1996).

Cryptococcal meningitis (Aquina et al. 1996), lymphoma (Gupta et al. 1993) and toxoplasmosis (Lanjewar 1994, Pujari et al. 1998), which affect the central nervous system, have also been reported. Multidermatomal herpes zoster has served as a useful clinical surrogate marker for HIV infection in the 15–45 years age group population in the country. A satellite epidemic of herpes zoster (Panda, Sarkar et al. 1994) has also been documented upon following the HIV epidemic in the young adult male population of Manipur.

Twenty-five per cent of the AIDS cases in Mumbai were diagnosed postmortem with acute encephalitis caused by *Toxoplasma gondii* (Lanjewar 1994). There has been substantial investigation of the spectrum of opportunistic infections in India with a number of autopsy studies (Lanjewar and Maheshwari 1994, Lanjewar and Wagholikar 1990). Almost all the autopsy studies in India have underlined the importance of keeping tubercular and cryptococcal infections at the top of the list of clinical suspicion while treating people with advanced stages of HIV infection.

HIV-associated Kaposi's sarcoma has been reported in low numbers in the country, the first one having been from Chennai (Kumarasamy et al. 1996). Similarly, infection with *Penicillium marneffei*, an AIDS-defining condition mostly reported from Thailand, has been reported in India only from Manipur (Singh et al. 1999). The clinical features observed in these cases were fever, anorexia, weight loss, hepatosplenomegaly and, more importantly, skin lesions resembling *Molluscum contagiosum*. The 1999 report extended the geographical distribution of endemic areas for *P. marneffei*.

The Evolving Picture of the HIV Epidemic in India

Although there is substantial regional variation, HIV is fast spreading beyond the groups of people it first infected in India. The progression of HIV from people observing high-risk behaviour to people without any obvious risk (the general population) in different Indian states has taken two to five years. Chennai has recorded an HIV prevalence of 4 per cent among housewives in rural settings (Solomon et al. 1998). As expected, HIV infection in newborn children occured in many of the states but surveillance did not reflect it. Leaving aside a very few NGO efforts, the benefit of neither short-course oral AZT therapy (evaluated in Thailand; CDC 1998) nor single-dose Nevirapine (evaluated in Uganda; Marseille et al. 1999) came quickly into public health practice in the country. It is worth noting here that within three years of incorporating into general clinical practice the protocol of administering Zidovudine (AZT) during pregnancy and labour and to the newborn for the first six weeks of life—which, it has been demonstrated, reduces mother-to-child transmission of HIV by two-thirds—the United States of America and France have shown a dramatic decrease in perinatal transmission of HIV (Mayaux et al. 1997).

The HIV epidemic is still evolving in India and the vulnerability of different population groups to HIV and STDs is getting better delineated with time. Long-route truck drivers have been indentified as a group at risk of HIV infection (related to female sex worker patronage when away from home) and also as a bridge population. The lack of social support for men who have sex with men (MSM) in India has made the characterisation of their vulnerability to HIV difficult. However, information in this regard is gradually being generated from the metropolitan cities of Mumbai, Delhi, Chennai and Kolkata, and even from Manipur where, until recently, discussions about HIV transmission revolved mostly around transmission among IDUs and their sex partners.

There are several plausible determinants for the observed heterogeneity of the HIV epidemic in India. Sexual practices in the general population and among IDUs, the capacity of sex workers to practise safer sex, which determines their vulnerability, injection equipment sharing practices among IDUs, and the existence of bridge populations between different injecting and sexual networks are some of the important ones (Panda et al. 1998). The types and extents of different interventions in different population groups, and the time gap between the entry of HIV and the launching of targeted interventions in a population group are also important influencing factors in this regard. The estimated number of people observing high-risk behaviour in a population and the chances of HIV transmission in and from them, the role of the socio-political environment with regard to safer sexual/injection practices as well as sexual and injection behaviour during the movement and migration of people differ widely across the country (Panda et al. 2001). The characterisation of all these influences and building interventions from there will have an important impact on the future course of the HIV epidemic in India.

The Wave of the HIV Epidemic in the Paediatric Population

The transmission of HIV to the paediatric population in India occurred in the early phase of the epidemic and mostly through transfusion of infected blood and blood products (Bhushan et al. 1994, De et al. 1990, Sen et al. 1993, Sengupta et al. 1992, Singh et al. 1991). A considerable number of thalassaemic and haemophilic children were infected through this route. An assessment of blood safety in the four major metropolitan cities during 1989–91 revealed that, while 88 per cent and 96 per cent of the estimated collection of blood was being tested for HIV in Mumbai and Delhi respectively, the figures were as low as 68 per cent in Chennai and 39 per cent in Kolkata (Makro et al. 1992). Although the situation has, of course, improved since then, India is yet to achieve 100 per cent safe blood transfusion throughout the country, the situation being more difficult in peripheral places—in rural settings as well as in hilly areas. Contaminated blood and blood products are still a matter of concern as sources of HIV infection (Indian Express 2001). Of the nearly 2 million bottles of blood transfused every year in the country, more than half were reportedly being supplied by people who sold their blood for money. Although the government of India has made HIV screening mandatory, not all blood banks comply with the law. The main issue is one of supply, as demand in this case exceeds supply. Currently, only 60 per cent of the demand is being met through official sources, and this has implications for HIV transmission

(Salunke et al. 1998). However, a critical appraisal of the necessity of blood transfusion in different situations is yet to take place all over the country, which could reduce HIV transmission to a certain extent, and 'component therapy' rather than whole blood transfusion is yet to be exploited to its full potential.

Kumar and colleagues documented mother-to-child transmission (MTCT) of HIV in 1995 (Kumar et al. 1995). The study recorded an overall vertical transmission rate of 48 per cent in the tribal women of Uttar Pradesh. A large proportion of non-injecting wives (45 per cent) of IDUs in Manipur has also contracted HIV through heterosexual contact (Panda et al. 2000). Vertical transmission is thought to be taking place in a big way in Manipur as well, the beginning of which was appreciated as early as in 1994 (Panda, Nabachandra et al. 1994). Maharashtra, having seen the progress of HIV in different adult population groups, also saw perinatally acquired HIV as early as in 1990. Autopsy findings showed the *Cytomeglovirus* infection in the lungs, adrenals, kidneys and large intestine, and fungal colonies of candida in the lungs, with pyogenic meningitis and abscess formation in the right temporal lobe of a child who died at the age of 47 days (Khanna et al. 1993).

Reach and Minimum Essential Quality

HIV is still spreading unabated in different parts of the country (see Fig. 1.1). Government, non-government and community-based organisations are working toward limiting its speed. A glimpse of these responses can be obtained in the subsequent chapters of this book. But the impact of all these interventions is yet to be evaluated on a large scale.

Control of HIV is closely related to the control of STDs, as 'epidemiologic synergy' does exit between these two, and improved management of STDs has been shown to reduce the incidence of HIV in some developing country settings (Grosskurth et al. 1995). In light of this evidence, the National AIDS Control organisation (NACO) has incorporated improved STD management as an essential component of the HIV control programme in India. But NACO also records that only 5 to 10 per cent of the people suffering from STDs seek treatment from government health care set ups (NACO 1999–2000). A more innovative approach is

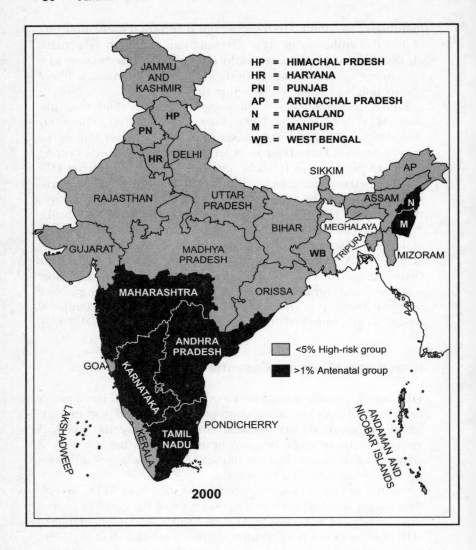

Fig. 1.1   The HIV Scene in India
[*Source:* National AIDS Control Organisation]

required to address the challenge of securing the management of STDs in wider masses in India during Phase II (1999–2004) of the National AIDS Control Programme (NACP) that the country has entered into. Research in Pune has shown that HIV testing and counselling of men attending STD clinics induces risk-reduction through consistent condom use with sex workers (Bentley et al. 1998). However this finding is yet to be corroborated by public health practices, where the standard of services is different from that of research settings, due to the workload.

The incidence of symptomatic HIV with multiple opportunistic infections is increasing in number all over the country, thereby compounding the task of the government in NACP Phase II. While a few symptomatic cases come to government hospitals, the majority either attend private clinics or stay undiagnosed. Attitudes of discrimination from the society as well as from a part of the physicians' community still exist. In response to the gradually increasing need for HIV/AIDS care, though with the simultaneous existence of an air of stigmatisation, NGOs have been able to reach out to people in need, but the needs are many. The State AIDS Control Society of Manipur supported the extended reach of a 'continuum of care' and the opening of hospices in 1999 to cater to the pressure of HIV/AIDS care and management (Manipur State AIDS Control Society 1998). Other states are trying to draw on the lessons learnt from Manipur as well as from different community-based organisations in this regard. However, the cost of treatment for opportunistic infections alone is enormous, leave aside laboratory investigation costs and costs for anti-retroviral therapy for HIV. With increasing numbers of symptomatic HIV infections every year, it is difficult to foresee how the need for care is going to be addressed in a developing country such as India.

A recent slash in the price of anti-retroviral medicines by pharmaceutical houses has been a welcome development (Subbu 2001, *The Economic Times* 2001). The Government of India also plans to withdraw customs and excise duty on anti-HIV medicines (*The Times of India* 2001). However, further transmission of HIV can be significantly reduced only by making anti-HIV medicines affordable and accessible to HIV-infected people and by effective scaling up of on-going prevention interventions aimed at achieving safer behaviour in the 80 per cent of the population with high-risk practices. Therefore, constant monitoring of the progress of the epidemic, evaluation and appropriate modification of the ongoing intervention programmes, active participation of the people infected with HIV in the designing and implementation of intervention, lobbying for further reduction of costs of treatment, as well as strengthening the general health care delivery system now appear essential for containing the HIV/AIDS epidemic in India in the long run.

Notes

1. HIV is the causative agent for the disease constellation known as AIDS.
2. 'Incidence' is the rate at which a certain event occurs, such as the number of new cases of a specific disease, during a certain period (*Dorland's Pocket Medical Dictionary*, Oxford and IBH, Indian Edition, 1995).
3. 'Prevalence' is the total number of cases of a specific disease in existence in a given population at a certain time (*Dorland's Pocket Medical Dictionary*, Oxford and IBH, Indian Edition, 1995).

References/Further Reading

Aquina, S.R., S.D. Tarey, G.D. Ravindran, D. Nagamani and **C. Ross,** 1996. 'Cryptococcal Meningitis in AIDS—Need for Early Diagnosis. *JAPI*, 44: 178–80.

Babu, P.G., N.K. Saraswathi, F. Devapriya and **T.J. John,** 1993. 'The Detection of HIV-2 Infection in Southern India'. *Indian Journal of Medical Research*, 97: 49–52.

Bentley, M.E., K. Spratt, M.E. Shepherd, R.R. Gangakhedkar, S. Thilikavathi, R.C. Bollinger and **S.M. Mehendale,** 1998. HIV Testing and Counselling among Men Attending Sexually Transmitted Disease Clinics in Pune, India: Changes in Condom Use and Sexual Behavior over Time'. *AIDS*, 12: 1869–77.

Bhushan, V., M. Chandy, P.G. Babu, D. Dennison, A. Srivastava, N.K. Saraswathi and **T.J. John,** 1994. 'Transfusion Associated HIV Infection in Patients with Haematologic Disorders in Southern India'. *Indian Journal of Medical Research*, 99: 57–70.

Center for Disease Control and Prevention (CDC), 1998. 'Administration of Zidovudine during Late Pregnancy and Delivery to Prevent Perinatal HIV Transmission—Thailand, 1996–1998'. *MMWR (Morbidity and Mortality Weekly Report)*, 47.

Chattopadhya, D., S. Kumari and **T. Verghese,** 1991. 'Limited Evidence of Human Immunodeficiency Virus Type 2 (HIV-2) Infection in Sera from Blood Donors Showing Positive ELISA but Negative or Indeterminate Western Blot Reactivity for HIV-1 Infection'. *Journal of Communicable Diseases*, 23: 206.

De, M., D. Banerjee, S. Chandra and **D.K. Bhattacharya,** 1990. 'HBV & HIV Seropositivity in Multi-Transfused Haemophiliacs and Thalassaemics in Eastern India'. *Indian Journal of Medical Research.* 91: 63–66.

Dorabjee, J., L. Samson and **R. Dyalchand,** 1996. 'A Community Based Intervention for Injecting Drug Users in New Delhi Slums'. Presented at the VII International Conference on the Reduction of Drug Related Harm in Hobart, March 1996.

Grosskurth, H., F. Mosha, J. Todd, E. Mwijarubi, A. Klokke, K. Senkoro, P. Mayaud, J. Changalucha, A. Nicoll, G. Gina, J. Newell, K. Mugeye, D. Mabey and R. Hayes, 1995. 'Impact of Improved Treatment of Sexually Transmitted Diseases on HIV Infection in Rural Tanzania: Randomised Controlled Trail'. *Lancet*, 346: 530–36.

Gupta, S.S., R. Joshi, D.N. Lanjewar and B. Kaur, 1993. 'Neurological Manifestations of HIV-1 Infection and AIDS'. *CARC Calling*, 6: 30–32.

Indian Council of Medical Research (ICMR), 1988. 'Changing Trends in Serosurveillance for HIV Infection'. *ICMR Bulletin*, 18: 39.

Indian Express (Pune), 3 June 2001. 'This HIV-positive Woman Got the Virus from Her Own Blood, Awaits Density'.

John, T.J., P.G. Babu, H. Jayakumari and E.A.F. Simoes, 1987. 'Pre-valence of HIV Infection in Risk Groups in Tamil Nadu, India'. *Lancet*, 1: 160–61.

Kaur, A., P.G. Babu, M. Jacob, C. Narasimhan, A. Ganesh, N.K. Saraswathi, D. Mathai, B.M. Pulimood and T.J. John, 1992. 'Clinical and Laboratory Profile of AIDS in India'. *J Acquir Immune Defic Syndr*, 5(9): 883–89.

Khanna, S.A., D.N. Lanjewar, P.G. Samdani and A.B. Shinde, 1993. 'Perinatally Acquired AIDS'. *Indian Paediatrics*, 30: 508–10.

Kulkarni, S., M. Thakar, J. Rodrigues and K. Banerjee, 1992. 'HIV-2 Antibodies in Serum Samples from Maharashtra State'. *Indian Journal of Medical Research*, 95: 213–15.

Kumar, R.M., S.A. Uduman and A.K. Khurranna, 1995. 'A Prospective Study of Mother-to-Infant HIV Transmission in Tribal Women from India'. *J Acquir Immun Defic Syndr Hum Retrovirol* 9: 238–42.

Kumar, S., S. Mudaliar and D. Daniels, 1997. 'Research Monograph on Drug Abuse and HIV/AIDS'. Chennai: Sahai Trust.

Kumarasamy, N., S. Solomon, P. Yesudian and P. Sugumar, 1996. 'First Report of Kaposi's Sarcoma in an AIDS Patient from Madras, India'. *Indian Journal of Dermatology*, 41: 23–25.

Lanjewar, D.N., 1994. 'Outbreak of CNS Toxoplasmosis Due to AIDS in Bombay'. Int. Con. AIDS, 7–12 August 1994; 10(1): 199 (Abstract No. PBO223).

Lanjewar, D.N., B.S. Anand, R. Genta, M.B. Maheshwari, M.A. Ansari, S.K. Hira and H.L. DuPont, 1996. 'Major Differences in the Spectrum of Gastrointestinal Infections Associated with AIDS in India Versus the West: An Autopsy Study'. *Clinical Infectious Diseases*, 23: 482–85.

Lanjewar, D.N., C. Rodrigues, D.G. Saple, S.K. Hira and H.L. DuPont, 1996. 'Cryptosporidium, Isospora and Strongyloides in AIDS'. *The National Medical Journal of India*, 9: 17–19.

Lanjewar D.N. and M.B. Maheswari, 1994. 'Prostatic Tuberculosis and AIDS'. *The National Medical Journal of India*, 7: 166–67.

Lanjewar D.N., and U.L. Wagholikar, 1990. 'Autopsy Report of a Case of AIDS'. *The National Medical Journal of India*, 3: 119–21.

Makro, R.N., P. Salil, B. Bhusan and S. Lal, 1992. 'Distribution and Trends of HIV Infection in Blood Donors of Four Metropolitan Cities'. *Indian Journal of Public Health*, XXXVI: 101–4.

Manipur State AIDS Control Society, 1998. Integrated Rapid Intervention and Care Project (RIAC), Manipur.

Marseille, E., J.G. Kahn, F. Mmiro, L. Guay, P. Musoke, M.G. Fowler and J.B. Jackson, 1999. 'Cost Effectiveness of Single-dose Nevirapine regimen for

Mothers and Babies to Decrease Vertical HIV-1 Transmission in Sub-Saharan Africa'. *Lancet*, 354 (September 4): 803–9.

Mastro, T.D., K. Zhang, S. Panda and K.E. Nelson, 1998. 'HIV Infection and AIDS in Asia'. In P.A. Pizzo and C.M. Wilfert (eds), *Paediatric AIDS: The Challenge of HIV Infection in Infants, Children, and Adolescents*, 3rd edition. Williams & Wilkins. 47–63.

Mayaux, M.J., J.P. Teglas, L. Mandelbrot, A. Berrebi, H. Gallais, S. Matheron, N. Ciraru-Vigneron, F. Parnet-Mathieu, A. Bongain, C. Rouzioux, J.F. Delfraissy and S. Blanche, 1997. 'Acceptability and Impact of Zidovudine for Prevention of Mother-to-Child Human Immunodeficiency Virus-1 Transmission in France'. *J Paediatr*. 131(6): 857–62.

National AIDS Control Organisation (NACO), 1995. Country Scenario Update, NACO, Ministry of Health and Family Welfare, Government of India, p. 14.

———, 1996. Country Scenario Update, NACO, Ministry of Health and Family Welfare, Government of India, p. 27 and appendix.

———, 1999–2000. *Combating HIV/AIDS in India*, Ministry of Health and Family Welfare, Government of India, pp. 1–36.

———, 2000–2001. *Combating HIV/AIDS in India*, Ministry of Health and Family Welfare, Government of India.

———, 2001. National Baseline General Population Behavioural Surveillance Survey, Ministry of Health and Family Welfare, Government of India.

Panda, S., A. Chatterjee, S. Bhattacharjee, B. Ray, M.K. Saha and S.K. Bhattacharya, 1998. 'HIV, Hepatitis B and Sexual Practices in the Street-recruited Injecting Drug Users of Calcutta: Risk Perception Versus Observed Risks'. *International Journal of STD and AIDS*, 9: 214–18.

Panda, S., A. Chatterjee, S. Sarkar, K.N. Jalan, T. Maitra, S. Mukherjee, B. Mukherjee, B.C. Deb and A.S. Abdul-Quader, 1997. 'Injection Drug Use in Calcutta: A Potential Focus for an Explosive HIV Epidemic'. *Drug and Alcohol Review*, 16(1): 17–23.

Panda, S., A. Chatterjee, S.K. Bhattacharya, B. Manna, P.N. Singh, S. Sarkar, T.N. Naik, S. Chakrabarti and R. Detels, 2000. 'Transmission of HIV from Injecting Drug Users to their Wives in India'. *International Journal of STD and AIDS*, 11: 468–73.

Panda, S., G. Kamei, M. Pamei, S. Sarkar, K. Sarkar, N.D. Singh and B.C. Deb, 1994. 'Clinical Features of HIV Infection in Drug Users of Manipur', *The National Medical Journal of India*, 7: 267–69.

Panda, S., L. Bijaya, N. Sadhana Devi, E. Foley, A. Chatterjee, D. Banerjee, T.N. Naik, M.K. Saha and S. Bhattacharya, 2001. 'Interface between Drug Use and Sex Work in Manipur'. *The National Medical Journal of India*, 14: 209–11.

Panda, S., S. Sarkar, B.K. Mandal, B.K. Th Singh, K.L. Singh, D.K. Mitra, K. Sarkar, S.P. Tripathy and B.C. Deb, 1994. 'Epidemic of *Herpes zoster* following HIV epidemic in Manipur, India'. *Journal of Infection*, 28: 167–73.

Panda, S., T. Nabachandra, S. Sarkar, S. Chakrabarty, T.N. Naik and B.C. Deb, 1994. '*Herpes zoster* in an HIV-positive 14-month-old Baby'. *The National Medical Journal of India*. 7: 63–64.

Priya, R., 1994. 'AIDS, Public Health and the Panic Reaction'. *The National Medical Journal of India*, 7: 235–40.

Pujari, S., R.S. Wadia, S. Bhagat and K.B. Grant, 1998. 'Seroprevalence of Toxoplasma amongst HIV Infected Individuals in Pune, India with Review of Cerebral Toxoplasmosis'. *AIDS res. Rev.,* 1: 10–15.

Rubsamen-Waigmann, H., M. Grez, B.H. Von, A. Pfutzner, G. Mahambre and J.K. Maniar, 1992. 'Two Indian States, Maharashtra and Goa Show Spread of HIV-1 and 2 Similar to Some African Countries'. The Second International Congress on AIDS in Asia and the Pacific, New Delhi (Abstr. No. B-334).

Salunke, S.R., M. Shaukat, S.K. Hira and M.R. Jagtap, 1998. 'HIV/AIDS in India: A Country Responds to a Challenge'. *AIDS,* 12 (Suppl. B): S27–S31.

Saran, R. and A.K. Gupta, 1995. 'HIV-2 and HIV-1/2 Seropositivity in Bihar'. *Indian Journal of Public Health,* 36: 119–20.

Sarkar, S., N. Das, S. Panda, T.N. Naik, K. Sarkar, B.C. Singh, J.M. Ralte, S.M. Aier and S.P. Tripathy, 1993. 'Rapid Spread of HIV among Injecting Drug Users in North-Eastern States of India'. *Bulletin on Narcotics,* 45: 91–105.

Sen, S., N.M. Mishra, T. Giri, I. Pande, S.D. Khare, A. Kumar, V.P. Choudhry, D. Chattopadhya, S. Kumari and A.N. Malaviya, 1993. 'Acquired Immuno-deficiency Syndrome (AIDS) in Multitransfused Children with Thalassemia'. *Indian Paediatr,* 30: 455–60.

Sengupta, B., M. De, P. Lahiri and D. Bhattacharya, 1992. 'Serosurveillance of Transmissible Hepatitis B and C Virus in Asymptomatic HIV Infection in Haemophilics'. *Indian Journal of Medical Research,* 96: 256–58.

Singh, Ng. B., S. Panda, T.N. Naik, A. Agarwal, H.L. Singh, Y.I. Singh and B.C. Deb, 1995. 'HIV-2 Strikes Injecting Drug Users (IDUs) in India'. *Journal of Infection,* 31: 49–50.

Singh, P.N., K. Ranjana, Y.I. Singh, K.P. Singh, S.S. Sharma, M. Kulachandra, Y. Nabakumar, A. Chakrabarti, A.A. Padhye, L. Kaufman and L. Ajellp, 1999. 'Indigenous Disseminated *Penicillium marneffei* Infection in the State of Manipur, India: Report of Four Autochthonous Cases. *Journal of Clinical Microbiology,* 37(8): 2699–2702.

Singh, Y.N., M. Bhargava, A.N. Malaviya, S.P. Tripathy, A. Kakkar and S.D. Khare, 1991. 'HIV Infection in Asian Indian Patients with Haemophilia and those who had Multiple Transfusions'. *Indian Journal of Medical Research,* 93: 12–14.

Solomon, S. and M. Ganapathy, 1992. 'HIV-1 and HIV-2 among HRGs in Madras'. The Second International Congress on AIDS in Asia and the Pacific, New Delhi (Abstr. No. B-345).

Solomon, S., N. Kumarasamy, A.K. Ganesh and R.E. Amalraj, 1998. 'Prevalence and Risk Factors in HIV-1 and HIV-2 Infection in Urban and Rural Areas in Tamil Nadu, India'. *International Journal of STD and AIDS,* 9: 98–103.

Subbu, R., 2001. 'Hetero Offers Anti-AIDS Drugs at $347'. *The Hindu,* Chennai, 15 March, p. 18.

The Economic Times (Kolkata), 13 July 2001. 'Cipla Cuts AIDS Cocktail Price by Another 39%'.

The Times of India, 9 August 2001. 'Government Plans Relief for AIDS Drugs'.

UNAIDS, June 2000. Report on the Global HIV/AIDS Epidemic.

World Health Organization (WHO), 1993. 'The HIV/AIDS Pandemic', *Overview,* Geneva.

2

AIDS in India:
The Government's Response

Geeta Sethi

March 1986. Six samples of serum in Chennai (formerly Madras) test positive for HIV. The then director general of the Indian Council of Medical Research (ICMR), Professor Ramalingaswami, writes to the Prime Minister of India, Rajiv Gandhi, informing him of the discovery. The prime minister, as was his habit, reads the letter at midnight, calls up the minister of health, waking him up to ask if he was aware that six prostitutes had tested positive for HIV. He further asked that a national strategy be prepared in two days. This resulted in an early morning phone call to the joint secretary in the Ministry of Health and, shortly after, the birth of the National AIDS Control Programme (NACP).

Such swift action seems to have marked the early phase of the government's response to the possibility of an HIV/AIDS epidemic in India, although it was only in 1985 that there was any realisation in India about the problems related to AIDS. There had previously been a mild curiosity in scientific circles about the suddenness of its outbreak in the Western world, and the overwhelming perception had been that it was a disease confined to the gay community. However, ICMR did consider it necessary to establish a task force on AIDS in 1985 and to start screening sera from high-risk groups at the National Institute of Virology, Pune, and at the ICMR Centre for Advanced Research in Virology, Christian Medical College, Vellore. In October 1985, the ELISA procedures at these two centres were standardised, and they were declared AIDS Reference Centres. This was the modest beginning of sero-surveillance activities in India. The National AIDS Task Force suggested that medical colleges in different states carry out clinical surveillance for AIDS among their patients. Serological surveillance of healthy persons from high-risk groups in selected areas was also recommended. The government banned the import of blood products that did not carry a certification of freedom from AIDS.

In 1986, the National AIDS Committee was formed under the chairpersonship of the secretary of the Ministry of Health and Family Welfare, to formulate, plan and implement a preventive programme. The other members of the committee were the director general of ICMR, senior officials from the Ministry of Health and Family Welfare, representatives of other government agencies and the administrator of the Voluntary Health Association of India, a leading non-governmental organisation (NGO).

Discussions and deliberations at this forum as well as outside of it led to the evolution of a control programme in 1987. The components of this programme were limited surveillance in areas and groups perceived to be 'risk-prone', screening of blood and blood products, health education and information. The director general of health services of the Ministry of Health and Family Welfare was made responsible for AIDS control activities in the country.

The National AIDS Control Programme included establishing a central AIDS cell in the office of the directorate general of health services, New Delhi, and AIDS cells in each state. The states were encouraged to have their own plans for AIDS surveillance. A network of laboratories and surveillance units was set up, including at least one in every state, and linked to reference centres for confirmatory testing. The Ministry of Health and Family Welfare, along with ICMR, developed a programme for human resource development through training laboratory scientists, organising workshops for state AIDS officers and a national seminar for clinicians through the Indian Medical Association. In addition to equipping medical personnel and services, the plan placed emphasis on awareness-raising and an awareness campaign on HIV/AIDS was launched.

The National AIDS Control Programme established in 1987 was reviewed in 1990, in consultation with the World Health

Organization (WHO). As a result of this consultative process a medium-term plan (MTP) for a period of three years was chalked up with an estimated total cost of US$ 20 million. The focus of the MTP was on the four identified high-risk metropolitan cities—Mumbai (then Bombay), Delhi, Chennai and Kolkata (then Calcutta)—and the states of Maharashtra, Manipur, Tamil Nadu and West Bengal. The basic strategy remained the same, with an added emphasis on interventions through health education and condom promotion among identified high-risk behaviour groups. Subsequently, in 1991, a comprehensive nationwide plan called the Strategies Plan for Prevention and Control of AIDS in India was drawn up. It had seven distinct programme components: strengthening programme management; surveillance and research; information, Education and communication (IEC); control of sexuality transmitted diseases (STDs); condom programming; blood safety; and reduction of impact. The Strategic Plan document had projected a budget of US$265.5 million for the five-year period, 1992 to 1997. The first HIV/AIDS project with a soft loan of US$84 million from the World Bank evolved from this document (NACO 1993).

1997. NACP completes a decade. The reported number of blood samples tested positive for HIV crosses 40,000. The reported number of AIDS cases crosses 3,000. There are reports that the actual extent of infection is much higher and UNAIDS projects that India is probably the country with the largest number of infected persons in the world—may be 3 to 5 million. There are indications that awareness regarding HIV/AIDS is low, even among health professionals and in urban centres, and the stigma and shame associated with the disease continue to be shockingly high, stifling the response to the epidemic which continues to be shrouded in denial.

What did this decade achieve and what were the stumbling blocks? While the government response was quick and a national strategy and programme were initiated with admirable speed, were we able to consolidate the advantages of an early start? Was the window of opportunity provided by the early recognition of a problem converted into gains that have impacted on the progression of the epidemic? What were some of the gaps between expected response and actual impact, and what areas of focus will make the government's response stronger in the coming years? These are some of the questions explored in this chapter.

The National AIDS Control Programme and the National AIDS Control Organisation

By the beginning of 1992, opinion at the top policy level within the government had crystallised in favour of a strong countrywide national programme to spearhead an organised response to the potential epidemic as well as to control and prevent the further transmission of HIV infections. The Strategic Plan document was used to initiate a dialogue with the World Bank. Negotiations were concluded by June 1992 and the programme was taken up shortly thereafter.

Programme Components

Operationally, the project involved all the states and union territories in developing HIV/AIDS preventive activities, with a special focus on the major centres of the epidemic. The five major components of the project were strengthening management capacity for HIV control; promoting public awareness and community support; improving blood safety and promoting rational use of blood; building surveillance and clinical management capacity; and controlling sexually transmitted diseases.

The budgets earmarked for these components were US$7.7 million for strengthening management capacity, US$31.1 million for promoting public awareness and community support, US$34.6 million for blood safety and rational use of blood, US$14.5 million for surveillance and clinical management and US$11.5 million for controlling STDs. The project, which came into existence in 1992, was scheduled to run till 1997, and was extended to 1998. Phase II of the project, 1999–2004, has now been launched.

Strategy

According to the planned strategy, the activities of the programme are to be implemented through the existing health infrastructure, the private sector, non-governmental organisations and mass media institutions. The Government of India coordinates the project, carries out major procurement and develops policies and technical guidelines. The actual implementation is with the state governments and NGOs, who are funded by the Government of India.

Programme Management

The National AIDS Control Organisation (NACO) was established as a special wing within the Ministry of Health and Family Welfare for strengthening management capacity. This wing is headed by a project director who has been invested with adequate financial and administrative authority to implement the programme. A high-powered multisectoral body (the National AIDS Committee) consisting of representatives of government and non-government agencies and eminent persons, and headed by the Union Minister of Health and Family Welfare, lays down policy guidelines and oversees the activities taken up by NACP. In order to strengthen the technical and research capabilities of the programme, a technical advisory committee (TAC) was established under the chairpersonship of the director general of health services, with eminent experts as members. In addition, a number of subcommittees were established to deal with different and specific issues, such as, control of STDs; blood safety; surveillance; quality assurance in laboratories; HIV testing; legal and ethical issues associated with HIV/AIDS; and operational research. At the state level, AIDS cells were established in the directorate of health services in each state and union territory, with total funding support from the Government of India.

Awareness Creation

A series of measures was initiated for promoting public awareness and community support. These included the preparation and provision of Information, Education, Communication (IEC) materials, services consultants and private advertising agencies, radio and television advertisement and publicity services, NGO services, audiovisual equipments, Management Information System (MIS) materials, training, workshops and conferences. The basic thrust of these measures was to use information, education and communication in a manner so as to effect behavioural changes that would contribute to the reduction of HIV transmission. The mass awareness programme was woven around (*a*) promoting safe practices, including safer sex, use of sterilised/disposable needles and other skin-piercing instruments, use of uninfected blood and blood products, and upgrading standards of health care, (*b*) influencing sexual behaviour patterns and (*c*) increasing the information regarding HIV/AIDS among people practising risky behaviour, potentially vulnerable groups, and health care providers. A careful plan involving mass media, interpersonal communication and focused health promotion interventions was drawn up for achieving these objectives.

Blood Safety

The existing legal framework was appropriately amended to make testing of blood and blood products for HIV mandatory, for ensuring blood safety and promoting the rational use of blood. In addition, and extensive network of HIV screening centres, known as Zonal Blood Testing Centres (ZBTC) were established in 154 cities in the country to provide free HIV screening facilities to all the blood banks in the public as well as non-government sectors (NACO 1997). Financial assistance was also provided to the states to upgrade and modernise the facilities available in all the blood banks in the public sector located within their territories. In addition, 40 component separation facilities are being established in some of the major blood banks so as to rationalise and optimise the use of blood and blood products.

Surveillance

Surveillance within the framework of the programme earlier had two basic components—surveillance of HIV infection and surveillance of AIDS cases. This has now been expanded to include STD surveillance and behavioural surveillance. Initially, surveillance activities for HIV infections were carried out through 62 HIV testing laboratories, designated as surveillance centres, and nine reference centres. A sentinel surveillance methodology was adopted in 1994 through 55 sentinel sites, and populations were screened for HIV prevalence and trends over a period of time. By 1998, there were 180 sentinel sites in various parts of the country.

Both, the sample size and the periodicity of surveillance activities were standardised. For AIDS case surveillance, a protocol was evolved under which all medical institutions participated in the identification of suspected AIDS cases. The referral hospitals were made responsible for the final diagnosis of AIDS cases and had to report them to the health authorities. This was supported by extensive training programmes for state and district health officers (known as physician responsible for AIDS case management, or PRAM). Both government and non-government professional bodies have been involved in this training activity as a crash programme.

Control of STDs

Under the programme to control sexually transmitted diseases, 372 existing STD clinics in medical colleges and other hospitals were strengthened through the provision of laboratory equipment and training of personnel. Other activities included the upgradation of five regional STD referral centres, provision of first-level STD care and counselling facilities through primary health care centres and general practitioners, and integration of STD clinical services in Maternal and Child Health/Family Planning (MCH/FP) clinics. As an integral part of the STD/HIV/AIDS control programme, an innovative campaign was undertaken to popularise the use of condoms and simultaneously upgrade the quality of locally manufactured condoms so that they conformed to accepted international safety norms.

Collaboration with NGOs

NACO sought the cooperation of NGOs in all the activities taken up for implementation. A comprehensive set of guidelines for the involvement of NGOs was drawn up and widely circulated. These guidelines were subsequently reviewed by state AIDS programme officers as well as by representatives of NGOs, and modifications were recommended. Some pilot studies and intervention projects were started with the help of NGOs in Delhi, Mumbai, Kolkata, Chennai and Guwahati. NGOs were also associated with training activities, IEC assessment studies, risk behaviour studies and the preparation and dissemination of IEC materials.

Social, Ethical and Legal Issues

Due note was also taken of the fact that as the epidemic progresses it raises several social, ethical and legal issues. A subcommittee was established to consider all such issues and make recommendations to the government. It was expected that these would be finalised by the committee during 1994.

The programme in India started with great expectations. There was, it was felt, 'a window of opportunity', which, utilised through timely action, could substantially impact the progress of the epidemic in the country.

Achievements

The government reacted fairly quickly to the possibility of an AIDS epidemic. Although there was scepticism in several quarters about the need for a programme, and the disease was perceived as one affecting foreigners and marginalised risk groups, the National AIDS Control Programme was launched in 1987, shortly after the identification of the first few HIV-positive cases. Further, the information received from early testing and surveillance was taken seriously enough to review the programme, and to formulate a strategic plan, in collaboration with the WHO and the World Bank. The government was prompt in negotiating a soft loan from the World Bank and in setting up the National AIDS Control Organisation under the leadership of an excellent project director. That AIDS was given some measure of importance was evidenced by the fact that the project director was devoted full-time to the organisation, and had no other charges.

Commitment to a multisectoral approach was shown through the establishment and composition of the National AIDS Committee, which included not only eminent government and NGO representatives but persons from diverse scientific and professional backgrounds, as well as persons living with HIV/AIDS (PLWHA).

The strategic Plan was a well prepared document and made provisions for focusing activity at the state level, since health is a state subject, to be implemented through state governments. The plan recognised the immense variations in culture and behaviour and also stressed the importance of working in close cooperation with local bodies, NGOs and community-based organisations, and through other sectors such as education, transport and tourism, and information, broadcasting and the media. The plan drew positive interest and commitment from certain quarters—international and bilateral donors, sections of the scientific community and selected NGOs across the country.

Some form of activity is now underway in all the states in the country. In order to expedite release of funds to various implementing partners, finance department personnel in the states were oriented to the programme and with the procedures required.

Surveillance to assess the spread and trends of the infection is presently underway in 320 centres across the country in accordance with a scientifically designed protocol. Testing is anonymous and unlinked, and includes high-risk populations, people drawn from STD clinics, as well as the general population at antenatal clinics. Blood samples, and not individual persons, are screened when blood is routinely drawn for other tests. This enables the collection of valuable data which is essential for advocacy and programme planning and implementation.

Given the importance of widespread awareness and adequate information at all levels, a decision was made to commission an advertising agent to handle mass media publicity. Some of the leading agencies in the country, known for their excellent public service advertisements, bid for the contract. After four long years of sorting out seemingly endless bureaucratic and procedural tangles, an agency was signed on to undertake the assignment. In the meantime, NACO produced an IEC training manual in association with Xavier's Institute of Mass communication, Mumbai; it conducted IEC capacity-building workshops for NGOs and state AIDS personnel and also assessed their IEC capacity to design appropriate training and materials.

NACO also negotiated for free time on television networks for HIV/AIDS messages. As part of reaching out to as many people as possible, and to provide a regular channel of communication to state and interested persons, a newsletter, 'AIDS in india' started to be published. There were efforts to mobilise the popular mass media, such as mainstream commercial filmmakers, through workshops to sensitise them to HIV/AIDS. Simultaneously, small and folk media, such as small theatre companies, magicians and musical performers, were also sought to be reached, to enable them to disseminate information through their performances.

There were some initial talks on motivating the newspapers and other print media to develop peer guidelines for stories related to HIV/AIDS, which would be sensitive to and considerate of the privacy and dignity of individuals, families and communities. Some packages of IEC materials for use in specific situations were developed in colliboration with NGOs, media/IEC experts and, at times, other donors. These proved very useful and were adapted for local use in various parts of the country.

A special effort was made to facilitate the involvement of NGOs, as it was recognised that interventions for HIV/AIDS prevention and control required dealing with extremely sensitive aspects of interpersonal behaviour and relationships, as well as with marginalised groups, such as, drug users, sex workers and men who have sex with men (MSM), who are unlikely to be reached by the government. The implementation of the programme was seen as largely the domain of NGOs and as multisectoral in nature. NGOs were sought to be identified in most of the larger states and were encouraged to undertake work related to HIV/AIDS, by integrating it into ongoing programmes rather than setting up exclusive AIDS-prevention projects. Training of NGOs in various areas, such as, basic information on HIV/AIDS, designing intervention, counselling and proposal writing, was also carried out. A set of guidelines for NGO involvement in the programme, to facilitate the application for and release of funds was prepared and disseminated. Simultaneously, efforts were made to equip state AIDS programme officers to productively work with NGOs.

There were some efforts at intersectoral collaboration, notably with the Department of Youth Affairs and Sports, through the 'Universities Talk AIDS' project, a peer education programme for colleges operationalised through the National Service Scheme (NSS). Talks were held and some activities conducted with the Confederation of Indian Industries (CII) and with the Federation of Industry and Commerce in India (FICCI), which sought to involve industries in the process. Initial steps were also taken through discussions with Indian Railways, the Border Security Force, and the Department of Women and Child Welfare on integrating HIV/AIDS prevention and control into their work.

There was a gross lack of information on sexual behaviour and, at the same time, popular conceptions denied the existence of multiple partnerships. The traditional ideal of a woman who was a virgin at marriage and completely faithful to her husband, along with the double standards that tacitly permit men to have premarital as well as extramarital sex, led to a situation where the existence of sex outside marriage was camouflaged so well as to be virtually invisible, and was definitely not discussed and acknowledged. Other risky behaviour, like men having sex with men, was also not acknowledged; it was seen as alien to the culture in the country and was hence not considered necessary to address. The ideal of sexual purity for women included 'innocence' of sex, which translated into lack of information, lack of ability and power to negotiate sex and lack of initiative in introducing the topic even with the spouse. In spite of these assumptions about sexual relationships, high STD rates, the limited research, and anecdotal evidence all pointed to the large gap between public pronouncements and what people actually did. In order to impact on the HIV epidemic it is essential to reach and impact behaviour, not merely produce rhetoric. Data on sexual and other risk behaviour and vulnerability was therefore needed. NACO undertook and supported several studies to explore patterns of risk behaviour in major cities in the country, and to identify opportunities for intervention. This was a bold step, as there was little research available on the subject, methodologies for research were also not well developed and there was a reluctance to take up serious research in this area. Conducting the research forged a new understanding and built trust and relationships that formed the foundation for effective intervention.

That healthy sexual behaviour is embedded in adequate information, understanding and acceptance of sex and sexuality was clear and was firmly supported by NACO. Concerted interaction with the National Council of Educational Research and Training led to the preparation of an AIDS education training package for teachers and teacher trainers. This package comprised a set of co-curricular activities, which could be conducted by teachers or counsellors. The package provided an acceptable way of getting sex education into schools and forms the basis for plans of including sex education in school submitted by 15 states.

Another area requiring urgent attention which the national programme attempted to address was counselling. The facilities and trained personnel available for counselling were entirely inadequate to take up the load and range of issues that counselling related to HIV infection and AIDS requires. Counselling is essential while revealing test results, in helping infected persons and their families cope with living with the virus, in moving towards safer behaviour by those who are infected and those who practise risky behaviour but are as yet uninfected, and for people who have doubts, queries or fears regarding HIV/AIDS. The plan envisaged training a cadre of counsellors—drawing on persons already in service and in a position to offer counselling, such as, health professionals in blood banks, nurses and teachers—in addition to regular counsellors, social workers and psychologists. There was a countrywide plan for preparing training manuals—one for training of counselling trainers and one which could be used as a self-learning manual for grassroots-level counsellors. A countrywide plan for training counsellors through five regional counselling training centres was also prepared and operationalised. This plan brought together academic institutions and NGOs as trainers and to provide practical experience.

Shortly after the programme was initiated, NACO realised that a major gap in the strategic plan was that it did not have a gender perspective. To expand the focus to include issues related to gender differentials, workshops were organised with NGOs and women's health activists, as well as with women's studies centres. These workshops identified priority issues, outlined a plan of action and defined research questions that would help address the special needs of women. A special issue of 'AIDS in India' was on the issue of women and AIDS.

Because early detection and treatment of STDs is essential for preventing the transmission of HIV, it was decided that the syndromic approach to treatment be followed. NACO prepared guidelines, comprising easy-to-follow flowcharts, to enable practitioners to implement the syndromic approach. These were prepared through a consultation with experts, and extensive training of doctors in the private as well as public sector on the use of these guidelines has been carried out. STD clinics around the country were upgraded through the provision of equipment and laboratory technicians have been trained and guidelines prepared for their use. Studies to assess community response, to develop effective IEC materials on STDs and to evaluate the syndromic approach were also undertaken.

One of the remarkable contributions of NACO in the first phase was its legislation regarding safe blood. Transmission through infected blood and blood products accounted for about 12 per cent of the reported cases in the country. While this was a high figure, theoretically, this was also the most easily prevented route of transmission. To work towards safer blood supply, NACO promoted a more rigorous screening of blood and blood products.

In what was a very bold step, the project director himself very strongly advocated for safe blood and appeared in court to bring about the changes necessary to include blood as a life-saving drug under the Drugs and Cosmetics Act. This meant that all blood had to be screened, that professional donation of blood was not allowed and that all blood banks had to meet certain quality standards to be licensed. Blood banks were provided the appropriate equipment and their personnel trained, to increase their capacity to provide safe, tested blood. More rational use of blood was strongly advocated, with special emphasis on doing away with single-unit transfusions. Making the most of every unit of blood, through the use of components rather than whole blood whenever possible was also emphasised. This remarkable legislation substantially contributed to reducing the risk of transmission through infected blood and blood products. It also enabled greater focus on the sexual route of transmission, an area that was difficult to address and often avoided through the emphasis on safe blood.

Condom programming, making good quality condoms available to all those who need them by improving availability and access, as well as educating people on the role of condoms in protection from sexually transmitted diseases, including AIDS, is critical to an HIV/AIDS programme. Although condoms have been distributed through the family welfare programme for decades, NACO had a long struggle to have them promoted for the dual purposes of planning or spacing children as well as prevention of diseases. The quality of the condoms being supplied, due to their specifications and lack of lubrication, was not suitable for HIV prevention as they had a high breakage rate and were not comfortable, especially for use during anal sex. NACO, therefore, worked towards changing Schedule R of the Drugs and Cosmetics Act to ensure more suitable condoms for distribution through the extensive network of the family welfare programme. The system of distribution was also made more flexible, with no insistence on noting names and addresses and no restrictions on the number of condoms given out per person. Social marketing of condoms was also stepped up. After lengthy deliberations, NACO convinced the Ministry of Information and Broadcasting that the timings for advertising condoms on televisions be expanded, and that they be promoted as dual protectors.

The programme encouraged the exploration and initiation of targeted interventions with high-risk groups and the more vulnerable populations for the prevention of HIV/AIDS. Some of these are very effective and are globally recognised as 'Best Practice'. The most notable examples are interventions in Kolkata, with sex workers and the sex industry consisting of brokers, regular partners, madams and clients; with MSM in Chennai; and with injecting drug users in Manipur and Delhi. The programme also took the first steps in setting up systems for a continuum of care from home to hospital, in Manipur and Maharashtra.

Another important step was the preparation and dissemination of hospital infection control guidelines. These guidelines are simple, practical and primarily seek to reinforce universal precautions that all health care providers should follow, irrespective of the threat of HIV/AIDS. Along with clear information on what to do or not do, the guidelines reinforce the message that HIV infection and AIDS do not require difficult or unusual precautions on the part of health care providers, but can be handled much like any other infection.

These 'achievements' did not come easily, as there had to be a continuing and intensive effort to garner support from those who should have been partners—state AIDS cells, allied sectors and sceptics within the government and the Ministry of Health and Family Welfare, who did not see HIV/AIDS as a problem meriting serious concern. Further, the gaps, lags and shortfalls of the programme were also great, and so, the achievements of the first phase, although hard won, paled in comparison with the immense amount of work still to be done.

Shortfalls

Although the strategic plan proposed was very good, operationalising it was not easy. The task was made more difficult by the failure of the programme to generate commitment and a sense of urgency at various levels. A decade after the first cases were detected, after the national AIDS programme was launched, and five years after the creation of NACO, denial of the existence of a problem continued. And this was so in spite of NACO reporting that over 66,000 persons had tested positive for HIV (NACO 1997—Monthly Update upto 31 July), and UNAIDS estimating the number of positive persons in India at 3–5 million. Somehow, there has been a gap in communicating with the general public and with key eminent persons and in defining the problem in ways which can be comprehended and accepted.

This denial of the problem was reflected in various ways that then impeded the progress of the programme. Staffing at national and state levels reflected the low priority accorded to the epidemic. Many officials held responsibility for HIV/AIDS work as additional charges and had little time to devote to it. Further, although a set of training modules for state officers to acquaint them with HIV/AIDS programme management was prepared, there was no mechanism to systematically build capacity or provide support and guidance when needed. Officials, therefore, had to rely on their own judgement, which often reflected popular constructs and attitudes, which were not always the most appropriate for HIV/AIDS prevention and care.

A strange paradox in the programme concerned money. While, in theory, there were adequate funds available, utilising these funds was extremely difficult. Either the procedures and the paperwork required or other barriers made the disbursement of money slow and hard. This constrained effective responses and frustrated those who were eager and ready to participate in the response. Their inability to release funds on time placed state AIDS programme officers in a defensive position vis-à-vis NGOs and other sectors, and strained relations that should have been mutually supportive and based on trust. The situation improved towards the end of the first phase. Procedural requirements were streamlined and rationalised, for example, participating parties were no longer required to furnish bonds to be eligible to receive grants. This facilitated the quick disbursement of funds and accelerated their response.

The government of Tamil Nadu, in an innovative attempt to overcome the difficulties in accessing and disbursing money, set up a society in 1994 through which funds could easily flow. This appeared to work well, and has been adopted by all other states and municipal corporations in Phase II.

Although there was an understanding of the importance of a multisectoral approach, and provisions were made to bring in other sectors through the national AIDS committee and through sub-committees, such as, the social, ethical and legal subcommittee, in effect, the programme remained largely a health programme, with limited involvement of other sectors. The importance of placing the HIV response within a larger developmental context is especially important in a country such as India, where vulnerability is determined by social, economic and cultural factors rather than by individually selected behavioural options. There is ample evidence that gender, poverty and lack of education and employment opportunities severely constrain sexual decision-making, and the option of practising safer sex is not available to women, to the poor and to those with little access to information and services. The socially compromised position of women, along with traditional notions of modesty, restrict sex education. Even discussing sex with one's spouse is considered inappropriate. The importance of proving fertility and producing a male child further pressure young women to have unprotected sex. Finally, the possibility and experience of sexual abuse and violence make refusing unsafe sex near impossible. The rising rates of HIV in antenatal mothers in some Indian cities, for instance, 4.5 per cent in Mumbai, Pune and Pondicherry, clearly indicate the inadequacy of present responses to enable women to protect themselves and their unborn children (NACO 1997). Similarly, migration in search of jobs, or due to natural or created disturbances, and lack of access to information and services result in vulnerability and in risky behaviours that require more than awareness and targeted interventions. These can only be addressed through larger macroeconomic and social policy interventions, implemented through a variety of sectors. Unfortunately, this kind of comprehensive response is still to come.

There is some hope that this may change, as the Prime Minister, Atal Behari Vajpayee, addressed a significant group of members of parliament in 1998, stressing that HIV/AIDS is a grave problem in India and that he expects every MP to play a role in its prevention and care programme.

The procurement and distribution of essentials such as blood bank equipment, testing kits and even condoms was uneven and often delayed, resulting in gaps in the continuity of services and activities. These delays demonstrate the low priority given to this activity. The delays further demoralised those working on the prevention and control of HIV/AIDS, damaged the credibility of the programme as well as undermined its exigency.

Another major shortfall was in the appropriate interpretation and utilisation of research findings. Early efforts, as is usual practice, focused primarily on the so-called high-risk groups. Testing and surveillance, for example, concentrated on sex workers and drug users. The conclusions drawn from these activities, which naturally highlighted the growing infection in the surveyed groups, strengthened the already prevailing stigma and negative feelings about these groups, and simultaneously reinforced the notion that HIV/AIDS is restricted to them. This fortified the existing denial of the threat of the epidemic and countered efforts directed at making HIV/AIDS everybody's concern. Confronted with this intensified denial, the approach that 'everyone is at risk' did not strike home and, in fact, made little impact. Research findings were often quoted without adequate reference to the context, appearing to make assertions that did not fit in with other data. Since data was so sparse, it was stretched to generalisations and statements not quite warranted by the study. This led to an overall discrediting of and scepticism regarding research rather than to an addition to information and a clarity of direction. Further, although NACO pioneered some very interesting studies, it was initially extremely wary of owning the results of these studies and in sharing them with interested partners. This is true of the studies of high-risk behaviour completed in over 30 cities in the country, and of the survey of prevention indicators. This created tensions with researchers, NGOs, local communities and donors, and was a barrier to utilising the information for advocacy and programming. This hesitancy in supporting research findings that are counter to prevailing cultural notions seems common and is part of the process of building commitment, understanding, and accepting sexuality and drug use. One of the major difficulties facing the programme was that 10 years into the epidemic and 12 years after surveillance started, there was still no consensual picture of the epidemic. There were widely differing estimates about the magnitude of the problem but NACO had not put together information from sero-surveillance, STD studies and behavioural studies to construct a picture of the likely situation. This hesitancy in making a projection was a large hurdle in efforts at advocacy. The epidemic remained hidden and invisible, and its denial continued to be strong. The reluctance to make a statement regarding the magnitude of the epidemic strengthened doubts about whether there was a problem at all. It also created situation where, in the absence of an official estimate of at least a probable range within which the number of infected persons is located, different people and groups put forward their own estimates, resulting in a wide range of projections, each denied by some group or the other.

The past few years have seen a change in the earlier unwillingness to produce and use data. NACO now includes the findings of the studies conducted early on in official publications. Further, research efforts have been intensified, with community-based studies on STDs, intervention studies to assess the impact of different approaches, socio-economic and household studies and behavioural sentinel surveillance, and other attempts to strengthen the understanding of the epidemic, its determinants and its impact have been carried out and the results disseminated. There is now a greater confidence about sharing results and about the acceptability and importance of such research, and its use. This has helped to guide the second phase towards a more evidence-based approach.

Although dissemination of information about HIV/AIDS was a primary goal of the programme, the overall awareness in various sections of the population continued to be low. The National Family Health Survey, 1993, recorded that 17 per cent of the women in the country had heard about AIDS. Awareness among key constituencies such as NGOs and health care providers was also not adequate. The low awareness was probably due to a combination of the inhibitions and the cultural sensitivities that hinder open discussion about sexual behaviour and related practices; it was partly due to insufficient attention to information that is perceived as not being directly relevant to oneself, and also due to limitations of the approach and the IEC materials used. The programme could not give adequate attention to the sociocultural context; it did not undertake an in-depth exploration of values, customs and social status as well as the different modes of communicating and how these impact on conceptions of sexuality. The programme, therefore, did not truly understand how all of these contribute to and play out in relationships, interpersonal communication, sexual decision-making and, hence, sexual behaviour and practices. The approach seemed to be based on the tacit assumption that the programme knew what was best, that it would tell people how to behave and its recommendations would be followed. Insufficient attention was paid to underlying developmental factors that shape and constrain behaviour, such as, poverty, gender and inequalities based on class and caste, and to accepting that individuals often have little control over their sexual lives. Similarly, there was insufficient exploration of the different idioms that work in different cultural settings and with different groups.

This is particularly surprising because, at one level, there was recognition of the significance of local context, of the importance of preceding IEC campaigns with formative research and the necessity of involving communities, the prime keepers of behavioural norms and peer influence, in all stages of the intervention process, and, at the same time, there was insufficient effort at local levels to create an 'enabling environment' that would facilitate and support behaviour change as well as the practice of safer behaviours through the exploration of different approaches. The programme did not really accommodate the range of existing perspectives and attempt to address each one on its own turf, starting with people's understanding, beliefs and behaviour. It tried to overcome the barriers imposed by cultural double standards and subterfuges by drawing attention to their existence, rather than by understanding them and working within the situation they represent, while simultaneously working with appropriate partners to bring about more fundamental, lasting changes in existing norms.

Looking back, this insufficiency can be partly explained by the need to fight too many battles on too many fronts, with a very small force. Some of the more complex and indirect aspects were allowed to slip through the cracks. The second phase recognises the creation of an enabling environment as one of the critical elements of intervention, and advocates for wider partnerships to make this happen.

Similarly, although a set of guidelines for the preparation of IEC materials was issued, there was not enough attention paid to monitoring the quality of the materials produced, and little to assessing the impact of different materials, media and approaches. Experience shows that most visual materials failed to make the link between what was seen primarily as a blood-borne infection, due to the emphasis on safe blood and information about testing, and the use of condoms. This caused confusion as well as a false sense of security that, if blood is not needed, or if only sterilised needles are used, that is adequate protection from HIV, and that condoms are then not necessary (personal communication with Sandhya Bhalla, CII). Given the large proportion of people unreachable by written explanations, a clear and simple way to explain HIV transmission is urgently needed.

The significance of the media in creating public opinion and shaping public reactions, and not just in giving information, cannot be overlooked in HIV/AIDS prevention. There was initially an effort to sensitise the media to the repercussions of the epidemic at the individual, family and community level, and to encourage mature, sensitive reportage, and an eminent media person was even included in the national AIDS committee. However, the sporadic, tentative advances towards the media have done little to genuinely inform reportage or editorial policies. The media continues to sensationalise and stigmatise HIV/AIDS-infected persons. For example, an article that appeared on the front page of the Lucknow edition of *The Pioneer* on 5 December 1996 showed a shocking disregard for privacy and confidentiality, and made generalised conjectures that were potentially damaging to the personal and professional life of the person the report was about.

There have been efforts in the past few years to strengthen media sensitivity through regular state-based workshops, monitoring media reportage and systematic attempts to liase with the media and invite them to substantive discussions to deepen their understanding of ethical issues. There have also been attempts to harness the positive impact of the media through an analysis of what works and what does not, highlighting the impact the media has had in the development field. Also, the media itself seems to have matured, and realises the significance of its role in the response to HIV/AIDS.

The importance of counselling in prevention, i.e., for changing behaviour, as well as in living positively with HIV, was repeatedly stressed. NACO developed a National Counselling Training Plan, with a three-tier system of training, and some mechanisms for supervision. This plan was implemented through five regional training centres around the country, and was supported by two counselling training modules, one for training trainers and one for grassroots counsellors. Unfortunately, there was a fairly long time lag between the development of the modules and their commission for use. They were, therefore, based more on the experiences in other countries than on the situation in India. More importantly, due to the time lag, the issues addressed in the modules relate more to prevention than to care and support. The modules and the counselling training, hence, were not synchronised with emerging and pressing needs. Further, the guidelines were not sufficiently stringent about whom to train, and trainers were of the opinion that several of the selected candidates were not suitable, either because they were too close to retirement, so that investing in their training was not sound policy, or because they had little opportunity to utilise the skills in their daily professional practice.

NGO partnership in the national programme was always considered important, and various suggestions as well as attempts at mobilisation were made to promote such partnership. However, the NGO guidelines formulated in 1993–94 were not effective to this end. There were difficulties in identifying suitable organisations, in reviewing and accepting proposals for funding, in the timely release of funds and in building capacity for work in the area of HIV/AIDS. Further, the model adopted to decentralise the process of involving NGOs, which revolved around the designation of one NGO in a state as the nodal agency for the state, did not work in situations where there was little trust and networking between the NGOs themselves. The guidelines were reviewed by state AIDS programme officers as well as by representatives of NGOs and other experts. The changes recommended were pending for about two years and revised guidelines, although prepared, were not widely disseminated. Further, there was a lack of clarity on the roles of the central government, the state governments and NGOs. Defining each role in a participatory and transparent manner, and such that each partner is comfortable with their required role and knows what to expect of the others, is essential for the smooth functioning of a collaborative effort. Linkages of mutual support and of building capacity, rather than of blame and mistrust must be forged between different sectors and at different levels of operation.

As NGOs' skills in counselling as well as their willingness and ability to partner with the government increased, some innovative models for the provision of counselling services emerged. Six

NGOs came together in 1998 to provide counselling at the STD clinic of a public hospital in New Delhi. In addition to providing a valuable service, such collaboration helps to maintain and standardise counselling and to train more counsellors.

Under Phase II, an NGO officer has been identified by each state, and the process of selection of NGOs made more transparent and streamlined. By now, more NGOs have built their capacity to work on HIV/AIDS and there are well defined models, well documented experiences and approaches to follow. The NGO effort has also matured considerably in these years.

The list of shortfalls should not discount the genuine efforts and commitment of several government functionaries who have worked with passion and tenacity in an extremely harsh environment to keep AIDS on the agenda and to try to make a difference to the lives of the millions affected and infected. In substantial part, the shortfalls are due to the lethargy of a system which takes much too long to respond, as well as the reality that initial strategies and activities were designed and sought to be implemented when far less was known about the epidemic and about how to handle the many complex questions it raises. At the beginning, commitment and capacity to implement programmes were also far less sophisticated and well developed than the epidemic required. In the time taken for those initial plans to be implemented, the epidemic raced ahead, but the situation now is dramatically different. In several states, the goal can no longer be prevention, but must include a much greater emphasis on care. In the first phase, the government response in India remained far behind the epidemic and behind what is known to work. It was not able to mature into a well rounded developmental initiative and to consolidate and build on the early advantages.

Major Gaps

There are still some glaring gaps that require urgent attention. The government must work in close partnership with other sectors in order to make any significant impact. While this has repeatedly been said, in practice, the government's relationship with NGOs, the private sector and even other sectors within the government has been adversarial rather than cooperative and collaborative, and NACO seemed to feel that sharing information and problems would show it in a poor light. While partners were willing to share the burden and do what they do best, NACO was reluctant to accept them as partners in the entire process of planning and policy-making and to give up centralised control.

Decentralisation was also recognised as crucial for an effective response, as it can increase flexibility and sensitivity, enabling the response to be in close harmony with local needs and prevailing knowledge and skills. The second phase has created organisational structures and procedures to institutionalise decentralisation. The state AIDS societies and the technical resource groups are examples of this effort at decentralisation.

Another gap is the lack of attention to human rights and their violation. Early on, the project did attempt to identify ethical and legal issues related to HIV/AIDS and set up a subcommittee. This led to some very fruitful discussions, and significant issues were raised. However, this effort was abandoned, and an important initiative was thus lost. The project now needs to start afresh, beginning with the lack of appreciation of ethical and human rights considerations within the system and the gaps in creating sensitivity to these issues in the present training of various cadres such as blood bank officers and STD treatment providers. There have been innumerable instances when health care providers, both within and outside the government system, supposedly trained to deal with HIV/AIDS, have refused treatment to, or have been negligent, rude and discriminatory towards patients; where the press has not respected privacy; where landlords have refused to rent premises to organisations of people living with HIV/AIDS; or where children have been denied education because their parents are HIV-positive. Two recent examples, a case regarding the right of a positive person to marry and the NACO stand on the arrest of NGO workers on the charge of obscenity, indicate the need for soul-searching and greater clarity on what the official stand really is, how multisectoral partners can step in at crisis points, and how far the programme is willing to move towards sociocultural change. These are just the more blatant, obvious instances of violations of human rights, which occur in many more subtle, insidouous forms, and at several levels. A strong initiative to address these issues is critical to create an environment where the basic conditions that foster the spread of HIV can be handled.

Closely related to this is the lack of attention and consideration to PLWHA as partners and key players in defining the response and in implementing activities. Again, while there have been efforts to support the coming together of PLWHA and form their own organisations, there has not been sufficient attention to developing their capacity to meaningfully participate in HIV/AIDS work. The efforts to create space to include PLWHA in policy-making and programming at the central, state and local levels also appear to be token gestures. Similarly, the various training manuals and guidelines, and the manner in which they are operationalised, do not focus on the human beings who are infected and affected and who should be the focus of interventions.

Finally, there have not been adequate efforts to, and no headway in, creating an environment where HIV/AIDS prevention and control can take root and progress. This includes the lack of commitment to the cause, the inability to form genuine partnerships, the lack of belief and faith in some of the approaches taken and hence subscribing to them in form but not in spirit.

The second phase of the national AIDS programme seeks to address the shortfalls of the first. The preparation for Phase II included intensive discussions with various partners—NGOs, the private sector, development partners, state officials—and an analysis of previous shortfalls. A serious attempt was made to develop a comprehensive policy, which has now been approved. The policy aims at an expanded and coordinated response to HIV/AIDS, with advocacy and ownership of the programme at every level being its hallmark. Prevention strategy lays stress on targeted intervention for control of STIs and reproductive tract infections (RTIs), and for condom use and blood safety, coupled with awareness campaigns in rural areas. An enabling socio-economic environment for infected people, protection of their human rights and provision of clinical care are other important aspects of this policy. NGOs and community-based organisations will be more actively involved in providing home and community-based care for AIDS patients. Multisectoral participation within the government and within the UN system and bilaterals is also advocated in order to synergise these efforts.

The plan acknowledges the spread of HIV from urban to rural areas and from high-risk to lower-risk groups, and tries to address both. It also acknowledges that the epidemic is not uniform across the country less than 5 per cent in the general population in the states of Maharashtra, Tamil Nadu, Karnataka, Andhra Pradesh and Manipur, where the infection has crossed 1 per cent or more in the general population; less than 3 per cent in states such as Gujarat, Goa, Kerala, West Bengal and Nagaland, where the infection has crossed 5 per cent in high-risk groups but is less than 1 per cent in antenatal women; and 1–2 per cent in other states, where the infection is still less than 5 per cent in high-risk groups and 1 per cent among antenatal women) and sets out different targets for different states (NACO 1999).

The main components of NACP-II are:

- Reducing HIV transmission among poor and marginalised sections of the community, at the highest risk of infection, by targeted interventions, STD control and condom promotion.
- Reducing the spread of HIV in the general population by reducing blood-based transmission, IEC and voluntary counselling and testing.
- Strengthening implementation capacity at the national, state and municipal corporation levels through the establishment of appropriate organisational arrangements, training and by increasing timely access to reliable information.

References/Further Reading

Correa, S. and R. Petchesky, 1994. 'Reproductive and Sexual Rights: A Feminist Perspective'. In G. Sen, A. Germaine and L.C. Chen (eds), *Population Policies Reconsidered: Health, Empowerment and Rights*. Harvard Series on Population and International Health. Boston: Harvard University Press.

Fathalla, M., 1988. 'Research Needs in Human Reproduction'. In E. Diczfalusy, P.D. Griffin and J. Kharlna (eds), *Research in Human Reproduction*. Biennial Report (1986–87). Geneva: World Health Organization.

Government of India and World Health Organization, 1990. 'Medium Term Plan for the Prevention and Control of AIDS in India'. New Delhi: Directorate General of Health Services, Ministry of Health and Family Welfare.

———, 1992. 'Strategic Plan for the Prevention and Control of AIDS in India, 1992–1996'. New Delhi: Ministry of Health and Family Welfare, Government of India.

Hawkins, K. and B. Meshesha, 1994. 'Reaching Young People: Ingredients of Effective Programs'. In G. Sen, A. Germaine and L.C. Chen (eds), *Population Policies Reconsidered: Health, Empowerment and Rights*. Harvard Series on Population and International Health. Boston: Harvard University Press.

Jain, A., 1998. 'Population Policies That Matter'. In A. Jain (ed.), *Do Population Policies Matter? Fertility and Politics in Egypt, India, Kenya, and Mexico*. New York: Population Council.

National AIDS Control Organisations (NACO), 1993. 'Country Scenario'. New Delhi: Ministry of Health and Family Welfare, Government of India.

———, 1995. 'AIDS Education in School: A Training Package'. New Delhi: Ministry of Health and Family Welfare, Government of India.

———, 1996. 'Country Scenario Update'. New Delhi: Ministry of Health and Family Welfare, Government of India.

———, 1997. 'Country Scenario'. New Delhi: Ministry of Health and Family Welfare, Government of India.

———, 1998. 'Project Implementation Plan: National AIDS Control Project Phase II (1999–2004)'. New Delhi: Ministry of Health and Family Welfare, Government of India.

———, 1999–2000. 'Combating HIV/AIDS in India'. New Delhi: Ministry of Health and Family Welfare, Government of India: 1–36.

———, undated. 'A Guide for the State AIDS Control Programme Managers for Collaboration on HIV/AIDS Programme'. New Delhi: Ministry of Health and Family Welfare, Government of India.

———, undated. 'Guidelines for Planning HIV/AIDS in the Community'. New Delhi: Ministry of Health and Family Welfare, Government of India.

———, undated. 'Revised Guidelines for the NGOs for Collaboration on HIV/AIDS Programme'. New Delhi: Ministry of Health and Family Welfare, Government of India.

———, undated 'Guidelines for the Involvement of NGOs in National AIDS Control Programme'. New Delhi: Ministry of Health and Family Welfare, Government of India.

Pachauri, S., 1995. 'Defining a Reproductive Health Package for India: A Proposed Framework'. Working Paper No. 4, South and East Asia Regional Office, Population Council. New Delhi: Population Council.

Priya, R., undated. 'Contextualizing AIDS: An Indian Perspective'. In M. Dadian and M. O'Grady (eds), *Cairo and Beijing: Defining the Women and AIDS Agenda*. Arlington, USA: Family Health International, AIDSCAP Project.

Vajpayee, A.B., 1998. Address at the Meeting on National Programme for Prevention and Control of HIV/AIDS. New Delhi. India, December 12.

3

HIV/AIDS Awareness and Control: The Role of Non-governmental Organisations in the Country

Ashoke Chatterjee and *Kusum Sahgal*

Beginnings

The history of HIV/AIDS action in India begins in the voluntary sector, with efforts being made by NGOs toward awareness and control at a time when official responses were restricted to denial. It was some four years after the Indian Health Organisation (now called the Indian People's Organisation) began its pioneering efforts in the red-light districts of Mumbai (then Bombay) in 1982 that the Indian Council of Medical Research and the Directorate General of Health Services launched a national programme of serological surveillance. This was to be the watershed event toward a national approach on the epidemic—the National AIDS Control Programme of 1987. Two years later, medium-term plans were worked out in collaboration with the World Health Organization (WHO) in response to national and international pressures. These influences were already making it evident that the challenge of the HIV virus would require a level of mobilisation well beyond the capacity of India's strained public health system. Yet, an umbrella organisation, capable of coordinating a range of policies and programmes directed at the impending crisis, did not emerge until 1992. In that year, the National AIDS Control Organisation (NACO) and the National AIDS Prevention and Control Programme (NAPCP) were established. Almost a decade of Indian experience with HIV/AIDS has passed since these events.

NACO

NACO's founding was not merely the turning point in Indian HIV/AIDS policy but also the point at which the essential role of non-government efforts became an explicit element in planning toward intersectoral and grassroots mobilisation. The NAPCP recognised the need for decentralised approaches in harmony with the constitutional reality of state (rather than central) responsibility for health systems. Official action was, therefore, to be targeted at state and district levels, while local action was to be carried out with the help of community-based NGOs. State AIDS Cells were made responsible for setting up 'empowered committees', on which NGOs were to actively participate. This was expected to help ensure that local responses reflected local needs and cultures, and to reach marginalised groups (such as commercial sex workers, or CSWs), to which only NGOs had effective access. As the behavioural implication of HIV/AIDS awareness and control became increasingly apparent, so too did the importance of the NGO route to people-oriented approaches, possible only through interpersonal linkages.

After the first decade of HIV/AIDS, with more than its share of chaos and contradictions, the rhetoric of community participation and decentralised approaches was firmly established. Moving from rhetoric to reality proved an uneasy passage, with nothing like the needed mission approach in sight. NACO, set up to function with missionary zeal towards participatory and decentralised approaches, became the casualty of political indifference which shackled its ability to act as a powerful national catalyst. Its carefully prepared guidelines were often blithely ignored at the most critical point of policy and action—state level decision-making. This

resulted in serious setbacks to NGO participation. In several
states, less than 10 per cent of the allocated funds were utilised in
certain years. With a few notable exceptions (such as Tamil Nadu),
empowered committees were either not constituted or left side-
lined. The low level of NGO participation excluded any sustained
experimentation with innovative approaches. Resource allocation
was a key issue in the perpetuation of conservatism, with NGO
ideas and action seen as a threat to bureaucratic control. While
NACO had clearly indicated, with the new culture implicit in its
guidelines, that India's overstrained health care delivery system
could not possibly cope with the numbers who would soon be
living with AIDS, the idea of government as facilitator rather than
controller remained largely restricted to paper promises aimed
getting at donor support.

NGO Responses

In such an uneasy partnership, NGO action most often began
with interventions aimed at high-risk groups. Condom promotion
efforts, such as those of the Indian People's Organisation in
Mumbai and Population Services International (PSI), were the
first and most prominent initiatives. The need for counselling
skills soon became evident. Christian Medical College, in Vellore,
offered early opportunities for developing these skills while
the Gujarat AIDS Awareness and Prevention Unit (GAP) in
Ahmedabad brought in the London Lighthouse to design counselling capacities suited to local needs. The growing implications
of the epidemic introduced issues of blood safety, outreach to
young people and the needs of particular high-risk groups. Much
of this was pioneering work and it included the mobilisation of
commercial blood donors (CBDs) in Ahmedabad by GAP, the outreach to schools by the Y.R. Gaitonde Foundation in Chennai
(then Madras) and the early work with truckers by SOS in Nasik,
AIDS Research Foundation of India (ARFI) in Chennai and Seva
Mandir in Udaipur. The condition of CSWs and their needs
became central concerns for groups working in every part of
India. NGOs learnt about the need for approaches that were
sufficiently flexible to cope with mafia oppression in Mumbai,
opportunities of mobilisation in Kolkata's Sonagachi district, and

encouraging 'condom enforcement' in areas such as Sangli, Maharashtra. Other experiments began with community- and home-based care, and then with protecting the rights of those affected. Following its defence Dominic D'Souza, a young man arrested in Goa in 1989 for being HIV+, Lawyers Collective in Mumbai became the first NGO to examine how its professional skills could be applied to the HIV epidemic. Other NGOs, such as PREPARE in Chennai, integrated the struggle for rights into their agenda for action.

Little of this work by NGOs was done as partners in a planned national endeavour, with identified roles and responsibilities. Rather, voluntary action was most often a response to local need or to personal vision. Direct access to donors in India and overseas emerged as a prime support strategy, bypassing erratic responses from official sources. While NGO achievements have been remarkable, indeed, sometimes heroic, the sector also indicated that voluntary action alone could not be the panacea. Simultaneously with bureaucratic obstinacy came the inability of many NGOs to professionalise as rapidly as the crisis seemed to demand. Many interventions were whimsical and ad hoc. Networking remained weak, with inadequate pooling of experience or sharing of scarce resources. Preoccupations with turf became evident and HIV/AIDS became an enticing bandwagon associated with big budgets and international exposure for some. In this charged scenario of NGO indispensability and challenge, the quality of the sector's response to HIV/AIDS demanded stronger management capabilities and more vigorous networking, and the everlasting hope of a more sustainable relationship with state authorities and NACO.

A Spectrum of Experience

In 1994, the authors were invited by the Ford Foundation to survey the experience in HIV/AIDS awareness and control activity of 19 grantees, some of who had been amongst the earliest interventionists in this uncharted territory. These were path-breaking efforts, tested in some of the most severely affected regions of the country. The learning which emerged from this survey and other documentation indicated important lessons of experience, underlining some effective approaches as well as an enormous variety of needs among NGOs. The findings offered directions of what could be done within the sector as well as from outside in order to strengthen NGO interventions. Three years later, a national convention of NGOs working on HIV/AIDS provided another opportunity to assess the earlier findings in the context of experience, as well as to better understand the prevailing directions of NGO action.

What Works

These studies revealed that effective functioning in the voluntary sector was often a reflection of individual leadership, a feature not unique to NGOs working on HIV/AIDS. Yet, in an arena with few models upon which to draw, and in which the possibilities of failure often appeared overwhelming, the physical and emotional demands on individual leaders made personal factors dominant. Charisma, however, was not enough; it needed to be tempered with the humility essential to foster trust and sharing. There could be few areas of endeavour in which teamwork was such an essential prerequisite for success. To enter and to survive in this sector, an established record of health experience offered another important resource of wisdom and experience as well as credibility in activities which were often without precedence. The risk of eager novices choosing HIV/AIDS as an entry point became obvious, more particularly as location-specific strategies came to demand mature experience in the culture of the particular communities being addressed. The need for research-based action thus emerged as critically important. Generating such knowledge also demanded a commitment to participatory approaches. Skills in listening and working from the bottom up were needed to replace prescriptions handed down from the top. Experience also indicated the need to avoid isolating HIV/AIDS as a separate compartment. Instead, it seemed essential that the epidemic be integrated into existing health structures and systems, as well as into other efforts at serving and empowering the marginalised. Mahila Sarvangeen Utkarsh Mandal (MASUM), an NGO in Maharashtra, for example, decided to treat HIV/AIDS as a health, social and economic problem caused by double standards in sexuality that had led to a lack of concern for women's sexual and reproductive rights. In Gujarat, GAP began to link its efforts with CBDs to the work of other service organisations more experienced in income generation and rehabilitation. Within an environment still apathetic, if not actually hostile, to integrated approaches, the challenge lay in developing management skills that could help NGOs select priorities from among the bewildering variety of jobs that needed doing. It became clear that training would have to be the catalyst — and of all the training needs, counselling emerged as the single most important and the most immediate.

Early counselling efforts revealed the critical importance of networking. Access to partners become essential to assist the requirement of a multifaceted response as well as to build the confidence and stamina of an emerging cadre of HIV/AIDS counsellors. Networking was also beginning to be seen as important to the communities that NGOs served. Collectivism among groups most affected (CSWs, CBDs and the HIV+) appeared as yet another need from the experience of several peer group interventions. In 1992, the Association for People Living with AIDS and HIV Infection in Pune emerged as the first group of its kind.

NGO Needs

The survey by the Ford Foundation indicated that the NGO sector's requirements began with the need for accurate problem definition. This had often proved most difficult in the absence of a reliable base of data and research. It required the generation of methodologies, models and benchmark studies that could establish indicators essential to monitoring and assessing project efforts. The implications of this for policy formulation on the national and local level were formidable, with NACO's, political difficulties demanding as a substitute a high level of professional response from within the NGO network. The capacity for cooperation, which was not yet strongly evident in the sector, was clearly vital to progress. Other capacities too had to be developed so that sectors and services could be effectively integrated and multidisciplinary approaches brought to bear on day-to-day problem solving. One was the ability to establish effective links with doctors and hospitals, working towards change with existing systems, rather than against them. To succeed, NGOs had to confront the general indifference of the medical community towards the HIV/AIDS challenge. This again underlined the need for networks that could help dissolve narrow definitions of HIV/AIDS as a 'sector'. In this effort, STD prevention demanded recongnition as a key strategy, with the provision of accessible, affordable and acceptable services for STD diagnosis and treatment strongly integrated into NGO interventions with health systems. Pune was the site for some of the most encouraging efforts at working with the medical profession, within and outside the official system, through the efforts of Health Plus and the Sevadham Trust.

Other management skills is short supply included that of fundraising, with scarce finance a prime reality among almost all participants in the study. This in turn demanded an ability to professionally manage funds. It also required effective advocacy and public relations skills, particularly in dealing with the private sector. Encouraging industry's support for NGO initiatives required creating a wholly new awareness of what indifference to the epidemic could cost in earnings and profits. Towards such management capacitation, NGOs began to move from individual and highly personalised approaches to priorities selected through team planning and networking. The threat of spreading already scarce resources too thinly over competing demands was ever present.

Networking was essential too for extending the learning from innovative experiments in the field, as well as to provide the stamina to cope with the immense human suffering. There was no greater management challenge than to attract and retain skilled young talent in this difficult sector, where stress was already draining many NGOs of some of their finest workers. Building team and individual strengths through training approaches thus emerged as a key priority, supported by documentation, data and reference resources, as did clearing-house services that could facilitate the sharing of information and experience among workers scattered over a vast and difficult terrain.

By 1994, communication in the sector had already acquired the popular sobriquet IEC—information, education and communication. Sizeable investments were apparent in IEC campaigns and materials. Most reflected a great, and often wasteful, diversity of understanding of what communication was or should be. The preoccupation with media products at the expense of behavioural processes was taking its toll on this sector of health, as it had been doing for decades on others. While donor enthusiasm for IEC was evident, the 'how' of it was often elusive. Some donors began to insist on research-based action, while the majority of educational, motivational and training material available revealed little understanding of research or communication skills. Communication awareness, planning and media skills thus emerged as major management capacities without which behaviour change, the essence of HIV/AIDS awareness and control, would be impossible to achieve. One of the first activities to highlight this need was that of addressing youth groups, a challenge many NGOs accepted as a priority. It meant surmounting the considerable social barriers surrounding sex education in India. The Y.R. Gaitonde Foundation in Chennai, Chitrabani in Kolkata and GAP in Ahmedabad were among those who contributed to a growing body of experience in developing communication strategies aimed at the young. All India Institute of Medical Sciences (AIIMS) recruited the celebrated filmmaker Shyam Benegal towards this need, while PSI's newsletter, Nexus, helped NGOs share developments in the sector with each other. To almost every group struggling with the demands of behaviour change, communication came to represent a major training challenge. It also became clear that media skills alone were not enough. The situation demanded strong partnerships with the social sciences. This link was essential to a strong foundation of behavioural knowledge that could inform intervention decisions, which would then require communication action.

These developments were also beginning to indicate the need to prepare care services for the HIV+, AIDS patients and for the special needs of drug-users—all areas in which the 'how to' was unclear. The states of the North-east emerged as a major concern, bordering the infamous Golden Triangle region—the world's largest supplier of opium and heroin. The Voluntary Health Association of India and local organisations such as Social Awareness Services Organisation, in Manipur, took a lead in this sphere while agencies such as Sharan and Sahara in Delhi focused on those afflicted by the growing urban drug trade. The special need to involve those experienced in rural health also became apparent as the epidemic spread deeper into semirural and rural areas. The beginnings of collective strength among CSWs, CBDs and the HIV+ offered another indication of the need for networks that could link HIV/AIDS efforts with those of activists experienced in collectivism.

What Could be Done

The HIV/AIDS environment may have appeared as one of unrelieved gloom in the mid-1990s, with a crisis of indifference at crucial levels of policy and decision-making. Yet, even then, evidence was emerging of the impact of national efforts; among them, the growth of condom acceptance and use, as well as the depressive influence of HIV/AIDS awareness on some aspects of the sex trade. Experience had been gained in understanding the variety of needs and circumstances that affected a spectrum of group and individual behaviours.

Research towards strategy development had quickened. There appeared opportunities for stronger involvement of resource institutions and for organised training. NGOs hoped to take strong advantage of the ongoing NACO survey of sexual behaviour in 65 cities. This was to be used to fine-tune existing programmes and assess the relevance of NGO policies and activities to local realities of need, culture and constraint. Available research and experience had made the requirements of several target group—CSWs, CBDs, truckers, blue-collar workers, drug users, medical and paramedical staff and the police—easing the task of programme design. Documentation of case studies could now not only speed decentralised approaches and strengthen capacities at the grassroots but could be a powerful support to the better training resources that were becoming available. Networks with hospital systems and medical practitioners were in place at some locations, offering opportunities as well as models for learning and for training. Directions and resources were emerging in counselling and care strategies, communications, collectivism, information systems as well as corporate support. Media interest had been initiated and media resources were available to assist NGO efforts, while a growing body of media material (albeit of varying quality) could serve future activity.

All of these developments also offered a stronger sense of reality and direction for donors sympathetic to this sector. Assisting stronger NGO networks seemed the most important contribution donors could make towards sustainability in the sector, along with capacity building through training and the strengthening of its research base.

NGO Networks

Following the 1994 study, the Ford Foundation encouraged the Tata Institute of Social Sciences to bring together the 19 grantees with other partners and activists, for a review of the pooled experience and its relevance to future action. A remarkable aspect of the gathering was that, for many, it was a first. There had been a minimum of sharing experience and learning among the grantees, even among those working in close proximity of each other. The knowledge that anxiety and stress were experienced by all infused a palpable sense of strength in many who had earlier reported being overwhelmed by the complexity of working on HIV/AIDS. Indeed, there was a sense of surprised reassurance that others too had been similarly challenged, had shared in suffering and defeat, and had found the strength to move ahead. 'Why haven't we met before?' was a question answered by the consensus that NGO networking was a paramount priority, made even more urgent by the chronic uncertainty over NACO's struggle for status and political acceptance.

A step towards organised networking emerged the same year (1994), when the Indian Network of NGOs on HIV/AIDS (INN) was formed, bringing together 65 institutions from 13 states. Membership rose to include 16 states when INN met for its second national convention, in Ahmedabad in June 1997. By the time the network convened again, in Kolkata in 1999 and in New Delhi in 2000, its membership had risen to over 100 institutions.

The INN Initiative

The 1997 INN convention provided a vantage point to review the patterns of NGO action over difficult years. While experience was maturing, there was frustration at the looming crisis of numbers just ahead, and the seeming inability of India in 'getting its act together' on a national scale. While neither the problems nor the agenda emerged as new, efforts at action indicated a new pragmatism towards problem solving. An ability to cope with uncertainties that had come to stay was clearly evident at this meeting.

In its deliberations, INN set out several priorities for grassroots activity, on the one hand, and for advocacy, on the other. Building and expanding counselling services emerged as the first requirement, a need of the greatest urgency, achievable within available and relatively modest means. Experience had underlined the importance of integrating HIV/AIDS within existing systems of voluntary action as well as of public health. Cooperation towards safer blood systems and TB control emerged as paramount priorities. Networking with and through other health systems/activists was also seen as essential to future care and support. Relatively little experience in these areas had emerged, yet the sense of urgency grew with the crisis visible on the horizon. Traditional Indian family practices were recommended as a resource NGOs would need to learn to explore, revive and strengthen. Research remained an area in which NGOs still found themselves greatly dependent on government initiatives, primarily NACO's 65-city survey of sexual behaviour. While these findings were still awaited in 1997 (as they were three years later, in 2000), it was felt that NGOs would need to build their own research capabilities so as to ensure that interventions are preceded by adequate questioning and reflection. Several NGOs had provided their services to the NACO survey, hastening the acceptance of research as a critically important capacity. This had also become evident through experience in such issues as gender, ethics and legal aid—aspects that were rapidly moving up the agenda. The need in HIV/AIDS action for much greater involvement of women's organisations and of authorities responsible for women's affairs was repeatedly underlined. Several NGOs, including Mother Saradadevi Social Service Society in Tamil Nadu, had carefully documented the impact of women's poverty and exploitation as a factor in the spread of the epidemic. Economic self-reliance was introduced as a strategy for HIV/AIDS control. Some participants called attention to panchayati raj (Village self-government) institutions as a new opportunity for action. Women's situation in HIV/AIDS was regarded a major factor in its ethical and legal dimensions.

Cooperation with women's rights and human rights activists suggested yet another networking strategy. Indeed, the 1997 convention strongly focused on human rights awareness that could offer encouragement and support to people living with HIV/AIDS (PLWHA).

Assisting such coalitions in their own networking and contact with legal, health and NGO systems emerged as a significant priority.

These discussions suggested that advocacy would emerge as a major NGO contribution to HIV/AIDS awareness and control— advocacy towards greater activism in the sector, better access to effective STD treatment, for condom promotion, towards a more rational understanding and use of HIV testing and at reducing PLWHA stigmatisation and discrimination while championing their rights. Effective advocacy across this range also demanded greater attention within NGO institutions towards better management capacities, including that of communications.

Then and Now

The journey from the denial of the early years to the AIDS band-wagon, and from there into the infinitely complex world of HIV/AIDS awareness and control, has brought perceptible shifts of emphasis in NGO interventions. Perhaps the most significant of these is the awareness today of the limitations of targeted inter-ventions. Inevitable perhaps in donor efforts to reach those most in need, this policy did also have the benefit of bringing together NGO and government teams in collaborative efforts. It also helped focus on the potential of NGO service and on groups often at the margin of attention and concern. However, targeted groups have also faced new challenges as a result. Public attention on efforts at service provision run the risk of accelerating the isolation and stigma that NGOs work to resolve. The case of truck drivers is an interesting case in point, one that has been the focus of a major share of NGO and official attention. An early barrier to health communication with truckers was the extremely risky work envir-onment within which they survive. Without any national approach to their personal and family security, 'safe sex' was hardly a mes-sage that could be expected to inspire them. Moreover, once the communication barrier was crossed, truckers found that national publicity of their role as 'carriers' brought with it acute social dis-crimination. Today, in some parts of the country, a young trucker must hide his profession if he is to find a bride. Migrants in urban slums, CBDs and CSWs were other target groups that have had to resist the impact of attention. Current NGO interventions, therefore, place new emphasis on raising a demand for change from within the affected groups, such as among CSWs in Kolkata's Sonagachi district. The need to address communities at large, within which professions and occupations exist, has also been a major lesson of experience—reaching societies along transport corridors, for example, rather than truckers alone.

Other policy shifts have included the need to transform the health delivery system as a whole, integrating HIV/AIDS into, rather than isolating it from, other concerns. This has led to new initiatives and partnerships. The most significant is the emphasis today on care and counselling, rather than exclusive preoccupation with prevention. With the end of the silent phase of the epidemic, AIDS patients have brought with them the need to develop systems of care and access to service that can be practical within Indian conditions. Working with families has thus become a major new focus of NGO activity. Another significant development has been the recognition of human rights in this sector, and of the need for powerful partnerships that can address issues of deprivation and inequity as well as of access to information. Networks are now emerging between those working in AIDS and other activists for social and political change.

These shifts also require NGOs to sharpen and acquire management skills in the relatively new areas (for them) of law and legislation (to address rights issues), the social sciences (to improve understanding of Indian sexuality) and communication (for both behaviour change and advocacy). The importance of replacing ad hoc interventions with those that are research-based is now widely acknowledged. Accepting a professional responsibility for using (and sharing) research findings with discretion has sometimes proved difficult. There have been instances of careless handling of methods and results, leading to confusion among activists and in public perceptions based on media reports. A warning sign came in the recent (2000) instance of NGO activists becoming the target of public ire in Kumaon. This led to their arrest for publishing a research report that many found offensive in language and content.

The problems often remains of who is to finance essential research. This was clearly a service that NACO was to provide. The behavioural survey undertaken in 65 cities almost a decade ago is yet to be made available, despite NGO involvement in the effort. No major new research efforts are known to have been initiated or published. More recently, in 1998, 15 Technical Resource Groups were constituted by NACO to focus on specific issues. This may be a sign of hope. Papers prepared by the V.V. Giri Labour Institute (on occupation-related issues) and by the National Law Institute have been well received.

NACO's image as a national catalyst continues as a source of uncertainty and anxiety for the NGO sector. It is yet to emerge as a proactive clearing-house or support system. A recent institutional change affecting NACO–NGO linkages has been the emergence of State AIDS Societies, as registered bodies with greater autonomy than the earlier State AIDS Cells within Health Departments. The new societies are meant to speed the decentralisation process, and to streamline NACO funding to the grassroots.

Whether these intentions will be fulfilled remains to be seen, and the decision that a government officer must lead the societies has been open to a variety of interpretations.

Conclusion

In the mid-1980s, the scale of the challenge inherent within the HIV/AIDS epidemic would have been difficult indeed to foretell. Institutions embarking on projects in the NGO sector could have been forgiven for assuming that they were adding another disease to their health agenda. The learning in voluntary action over the next years was that HIV/AIDS brings together, perhaps like nothing else, every possible dimension of Indian life and suffering— social, economic, political, medical. Until a few years ago, there was a real danger that this complexity would overwhelm those working outside established systems.

In the absence of strong national policy or support, NGOs seemed often on the verge of burning out. Today their ability to serve and survive has been demonstrated. There is a palpable stirring of confidence. Some of this may derive from emerging networks of cooperation and perhaps even from the realisation that while so much more could have been achieved if the government's role had been less erratic, there is unmistakable evidence of self-reliance that works. While circumstances often forced self-reliance on the NGO community, within which necessity has had to be the mother of innovation, this can be registered as its modest but significant achievement in the alleviation of a new Indian suffering. Taking the effort to scale is the challenge ahead.

References/Further Reading

Asthana, Sheena, 1996. 'AIDS-related Policies, Legislation and Programme Implementation in India'. *Health Policy and Planning,* 11(2): 184–97. Oxford University Press.

Chatterjee, Ashoke, 1991. 'AIDS in India'. *AIDS Watch,* 13: 3–7.

Chatterjee, Ashoke and **Kusum Sahgal,** 1994. 'HIV/AIDS Awareness & Control'. A survey for the Ford Foundation, New Delhi.

International Society for Research on Civilization Diseases and on Environment (India), 1996. 'Responsible Health Behaviour: Citizen's Role'. Ahmedabad: ISCRCDE.

Narain, Jai P. and **A. Jha,** 1997. 'NGOs & AIDS'. New Delhi: WHO Regional Office for South-East Asia.

National AIDS Control Organisation, 1996. 'National AIDS Control Programme in India. Country Scenario: An Update'. New Delhi: Ministry of Health and Family Welfare, Government of India.

NEXUS, 1996/1997. A publication of Population Services International, New Delhi.

NGO-AIDS Cell, Centre for Community Medicine, 1995.*Directory of Non-governmental Organisations Working for AIDS Prevention.* New Delhi. All India Institute of Medical Sciences.

Shreedhar, Jaya and **Anthony Colaco,** 1996. 'Broadening the Front'. New Delhi: ActionAid, British Council, UNDP.

4

HIV Risk Behaviour and the Sociocultural Environment in India

Ravi K. Verma and Tarun K. Roy

A well known but little understood fact is the complex relationship between sociocultural environments and the spread of HIV/AIDS. Information, education and communication (IEC) efforts and behavioural change strategies about practising safer sex cannot produce the desirable effects if these efforts are not contextualised within the cultural and social environments that sustain and often promote the risky behaviours (Mane and Maitra 1992). In this chapter we will attempt to review the current state of knowledge on issues relating to the socio-economic and cultural environment in which the HIV/AIDS epidemic is breeding in India.

The Changing Scenario of HIV/AIDS in India

The spread of HIV in the South Asian region began in the mid-1980s, with the identification of the first case in 1986 in Chennai (then Madras), India. Although, the infection was initially viewed as being primarily concentrated among people practising high-risk behaviour, by the late 1990s it became evident that the transmission of HIV/AIDS among several subgroups of the general population in India was increasing, in some cases, with great speed.

More crucially, these subgroups did not necessarily display high-risk behaviour. This observation is substantiated by the round of sentinel surveillance (NACO 1999–2000), which shows that in at least six states, more than 1 per cent of the pregnant women in urban areas are now infected by HIV. India's rural areas, home to 73 per cent of the country's 1 billion people, were earlier believed to be relatively free of the epidemic. New studies show that at least in some areas HIV has become common in villages as well. A survey of randomly selected houses in Tamil Nadu showed that 2.1 per cent of the adult population living in the countryside had HIV, as compared to 0.7 per cent of the urban population. The epidemic continues to shift towards women and young people; 21 per cent of all HIV infections are estimated to be among women, with the female–male ratio of infection sharply increasing (Gangakhedkar et al. 1997). Increased HIV infections in young women in the reproductive age group is accompanied by an increase in vertical transmission and paediatric AIDS.

A majority of the women do not have any risk factor other than being married to their husbands. Data from sentinel surveillance point to a rapid evolution of the epidemic, especially in the southern and western parts of India. Andhra Pradesh and Karnataka have now overtaken Tamil Nadu to join Maharashtra as the states with the highest prevalence of HIV. A distinct but continuing epidemic among injecting drug users in Manipur has been documented to spread to their spouses—45 per cent of the non-injecting wives of injecting drug users (IDUs) testing HIV-positive through hetero-sexual transmission from their husbands (Panda et al. 2000). The major northern states still report very low levels of HIV. Their vulnerability to the epidemic, due to male migration, adverse gender norms and weak infrastructure, however, makes action in these states critical to impact the future path of the epidemic. Given its large and increasing population, India is soon expected to have the largest concentration of AIDS-affected individuals in the world, if the current rate of transmission continues.

Some recent facts about the HIV epidemic in India

- HIV prevalence in India doubled over the last four years, resulting in India having the highest number of HIV infections in the world—an estimated 3.9 million.

- In Andhra Pradesh, Tamil Nadu, Karnataka, Maharashtra, Manipur and Nagaland, HIV prevalence has reached over 1 per cent among women attending antenatal clinics. In most other parts of the country, the overall levels of HIV are still low, though male migration, adverse gender norms and weak infrastructure make almost all states vulnerable to the rapid spread of the infection.

- Eighty-nine per cent of the reported HIV cases are in the sexually active and economically productive age group of 18–40 years. Over 50 per cent of all new infections take place among young adults below the age of 25 years. Twenty-one per cent of new HIV infections are among women—a majority of who do not have any other risk factor than being married to their husbands.

- Eighty-three per cent of HIV infections in the reported cases of AIDS are through sexual transmission, 2 per cent through perinatal transmission, 4 per cent through injecting drug use, another 4 per cent through blood transfusion and blood product infusion, and the remaining 7 per cent is categorised as 'others'.

Socio-economic and Cultural Environment

Three sets of factors strongly influenced the course of the emerging HIV/AIDS epidemic in different parts of India—sexual contact, contaminated blood and patterns of injection drug use. However, the complex epidemic that has emerged in India is primarily one of heterosexual transmission, fuelled by an active sex industry and interacting with less studied patterns of bisexual and/or injecting behaviour. These factors are aggravated due to several social, economic and cultural factors.

Poverty and Low Economic Status
Create Conditions for the Spread of HIV/AIDS

Over 300 million people, or 36 per cent of the population, in India live below the poverty line. The average literacy rate in India is 39.4 per cent for women and 66.7 per cent for men. India has a large and thriving sex industry, estimated to number around 100,000 workers in each of the metropolitan cities (Verma et al. 1999). Due to the clandestine nature of the trade, the majority of sex workers lack legal provisions, suffer discrimination and have few means of protecting themselves. The poor and uneducated in a society are more likely to contract sexually transmitted diseases (STDs) and other infections since they are deprived of the right to information on risk behaviour, are too illiterate to understand prevention messages and have less access to quality services.

Untreated STDs Raise the Risk of
HIV Infection Per Sexual Exposure

India has a very high prevalence of sexually transmitted diseases and studies show that people with current or past STDs are two to nine times more likely to get infected with HIV. The lesions caused by untreated ulcerative STDs such as herpes, syphilis and chancroid provide an easy entry and transmission portal for HIV. Based on available data, it is estimated that the annual incidence of STDs in India may be as high as 5 per cent of the population, with over 40 million new infections per year (Salunke et al. 1998). STD baseline surveys conducted in Chennai and Jaipur, as well as among sex workers in Kolkata and in a rural area of Tamil Nadu, reveal that STDs are clearly not an exclusively urban problem; prevalence rates for urban populations range from 1.2 per cent to 10 per cent and go up to 7 per cent for rural populations (Rodrigues et al. 1995). According to a recent report (Mehendale 1998), one in every five males and one in every two sex workers coming to an STD clinic in Pune was found to be HIV+. Similar rates of infection are being reported in STD clinics in other parts of the country.

Double Standards of Morality and Gender Norms

Discriminatory standards of morality and gender norms, leading to conditions where women are denied the same rights as men, are important factors in the spread of HIV/AIDS. Women have little or no control over decisions relating to their sexuality, over the sexual behaviour of their male partners or the use of condoms for the prevention of pregnancy or STD/AIDS. Twenty-one per cent of all HIV infections is now estimated to be in women (Gangakhedkar et al. 1997) and the number of those infected is on the rise, with an accompanying increase in vertical transmission and paediatric AIDS. Antenatal clinics in all major cities are reporting increasing levels of HIV infection.

Population Mobility

Population mobility is a key factor in the spread of HIV in India. Limited employment opportunities force people to move from rural to urban areas, from one state to another and from one country to another. There are over 180 million migrant workers in India (Hira et al. 1998), many of who are single men or men who live apart from their wives and families. Other mobile populations such as members of the armed forces and long-route truck drivers are more likely to have unsafe sex. It is this high mobility of the male population that has brought the virus to rural areas. Migrant men comprise 30–40 per cent of the population of large cities, where they also account for much of the clientele of 'red light' areas. In a study of 5,722 male truck drivers in Assam, 82 per cent reported regular sex with female sex workers along the national highways, and none of the men used condoms regularly; 15 per cent reported a history of sex with men; 36 per cent had been treated for STDs; 40 per cent used cannabis and 2.4 per cent had injected heroin. A recent study conducted in Wazirpur Industrial Area, near New Delhi, reports a high prevalence of paid multi-partner sex and low condom use among industrial workers, many of who were away from their families (Singh 1999). HIV infection among workers in two industrial units in Mumbai was found to be 3 per cent and 2.5 per cent respectively in 1996 (Hira et al. 1998). Crisis situations in the Northeast, where IDUs had to move away from their respective home towns following violent ethnic clashes during 1997–98, has also been documented while migration disrupted HIV/AIDS intervention activities. This also forced women drug users to take up sex work, thus highlighting the link between political unrest and HIV/AIDS in India (Panda 2001).

Rapid Urbanisation

Economic growth has led to rapid urbanisation, which in turn has resulted in large slum populations and an increase in categories of unorganised labour such as construction workers, casual land-less labourers and child workers. In 1996, some 100 million people were estimated to be living in urban slums, a figure that was expected to rise to 110 million by 2001 (Pandav et al. 1997). Two-thirds of these are children, youth and women who are less literate, lack basic knowledge of safe health practices and have little or no access to information or to health and other supportive services. Poverty, ignorance and violation of basic rights in these areas create the conditions which facilitate the spread of HIV.

Sexual Behaviour vis-à-vis Prevention Knowledge and Practice

Behavioural studies conducted by NACO show that sexual risk practice is well established in India (NACO 1997). Unprotected sex and a high rate of partner exchange through casual and commercial sex is the driving force behind the rapid spread of HIV among female sex workers and their clients, who then pass it on to their wives. A study in Pune clearly illustrates this situation, which is common to many societies. Of a sample of nearly 400 women attending the city's STI clinics, almost all of who had contact with partners with sexually transmitted infections, at least 25 per cent were infected with an STD and 13.6 per cent tested positive for HIV. Ninety-three per cent of these women were married and 91 per cent had never had sex with anyone but their husbands (Mehendale et al. 1998). A 1995 study by NACO also revealed low knowledge of prevention practices, especially in rural areas, and that even where knowledge levels were high, as in some of the major cities, misconceptions had still not been dispelled. On the other hand, several constraints in condom use, independent of each other, such as the belief that condom use leads to a loss of pleasure, cultural sensitivity, its association with birth control, the powerlessness of women in ensuring safety and the lack of assurance of quality, have all led to low condom use, especially with non-regular partners (Rangaiyan and Verma 2001).

Reluctance to Address Sex and Sex-related Issues

The denial of the existence of risk behaviour, in particular among young people, facilitates the spread of HIV and other STDs in them. In general, the topic of sex is taboo and is closely linked to morals and promiscuity. All these lead to inadequate policy support for sex education in schools and for out-of-school youth, as well as to a denial of the right to information and services. Out of the 121 million Indian children of primary school age, around 109 million are currently in school. But by the time sex education enters the curriculum, half of all the boys and almost 60 per cent of the girls have dropped out of school.

Male-to-male Sex

Male-to-male sex is morally proscribed behaviour, forcing men who have sex with men (MSM) underground. Studies among relatively small samples of MSM in Mumbai in the early 1990s recorded levels of HIV infection ranging between 3 and 15 per cent (Nag 1996). However, because homosexuality is socially unacceptable in India, many of these men are married or have regular female partners. In one study among truck dirvers, between a third and a half of the respondents said that they had had oral or anal sex with other men, and that they also had sex with women (Rao et al. 1994).

Injection Drug Use

Sharing of injecting equipment is potentially a major route for HIV transmission, as evidenced by the extremely high prevalence of HIV in north-east India and in some of the major cities. Some sites in Manipur have reported prevalence as high as 70 per cent and a 1999 study in New Delhi found 45 per cent of the injectors linked to a treatment centre to be HIV+ (Sharan 1998). The sexual and IDU networks may include the same members, i.e., IDUs who share needles may also trade sex for money (for drugs) and thereby increase their chances of infection. Infection has also been known to spread to the non-injecting sexual partners of IDUs; some 1.25 per cent of pregnant women (visiting ANCs) tested positive in Manipur in 1998 (Shourie 2000).

It must be noted that injecting drug use is seen as an offence by the law and enforcement personnel, which drives IDUs underground, preventing them from accessing information and support services for protection from infection. Moreover, sudden non-availability of brown sugar in the market due to stringent drug seizure has been found to be associated with an increase in injecting drug use, which highlights the relationship between environmental change and the increased vulnerability of a group of people to HIV/AIDS and other blood-borne infections (Panda 1997).

Young Populations

India has a large population of young people—about 400 million below the age of 18 years. Studies and field experience provide evidence of the early onset of sexual activity and the low levels of awareness among young people (Pelto et al. 2000). There is also a comparatively large population of children living in difficult circumstances, such as street children and child labourers, many of whom are vulnerable to sexual abuse. As the epidemic matures, there is an increasing pool of potential sexual partners who are already infected. This is true for young men, who, in many countries, tend to have their first sexual encounters with sex workers, and also for young women, who might be forced through circumstances to have sex with older men.

Young people are also made more vulnerable to HIV by certain taboos, ideologies and social norms. This is particularly the case when young people are denied knowledge and skills on sexual and reproductive matters, barred from reproductive health services, including HIV prevention and STD care and counselling, and ostracised if attracted to the same sex. Adolescents are generally left alone to deal with the biological and social transformation of adolescence, often with no caring adults to talk to.

Discrimination and the Curtailing of Human Rights

Discrimination against and the denial of human rights to women, children, marginalised populations, such as street children, female sex workers, sexual minority populations, and men who have sex with men have resulted in their lack of access to information and acceptable services. This also heightens the risk of infection and promotes the further spread of the virus. Discrimination against people living with HIV/AIDS (PLWHA) forces them to remain socially invisible and to deny their status to protect themselves from social ostracism from their own families and communities. Many of the affected are struggling to cope, unable to come out and avail services because when they do, they are rejected by the people who should help—the health care service providers. Reports of hospital-based discrimination and stigmatisation are widely documented and anecdotal evidence of employment-related discrimination has also begun to emerge. The Indian Supreme Court has ruled that the people who are HIV+ must inform future spouses of their infection. In a judgement made public, the court also said that hospitals could not be charged with violating medical ethics when they disclosed the HIV+ status of an infected individual to a person he or she intended to marry (Mudur 1998). The net result of this discrimination and lack of visibility of PLWHA is the perpetuation of a social climate of fear and misconceptions and the unchecked spread of HIV.

Low Level of Knowledge and Awareness

Given the increasing vulnerability of women and children in the general population, the National Family Health Survey-2 (NFHS-2) of 1998 had included a set of questions on knowledge of AIDS and AIDS prevention for every married women of the age group 15–49 years. It is worth noting that NACO spends about 34 per cent of its funds on information, education and communication (IEC) activities. However, several small-scale studies as well as

NFHS-2 reveal that the general public is quite ignorant about HIV/AIDS and ways to aviod infection. The NFHS data suggests that 60 per cent of ever-married women between the ages of 15 and 49 years had never heard of AIDS, and of those who had, one-third did not know how to avoid getting it. Of course, there is very wide variation in knowledge across social and economic lines. While 70 per cent of the urban women in the study had heard about AIDS, only 30 per cent of the rural women reported such awareness. A few in-depth studies have confirmed that while knowledge depends on economic factors such as income, it also depends on a number of sociocultural factors such as age, marital status and state of origin (Basu et al. 1995). The young, unmarried male from Delhi, for example, was much more correctly informed than his more conservative, older, married counterpart from other parts of northern India.

Regarding sources of information, NFHS-2 showed that television was most important source of information about AIDS among ever-married women (79 per cent). Among women who said that something could be done to prevent AIDS, the most commonly mentioned ways of avoiding AIDS were having only one sex partner (40 per cent) and avoiding used needles or using clean needles (30 per cent). In contrast is the information that a significant proportion of married women in Manipur, Pune and other places in India have become infected with HIV through monogamous relationships with their husbands. NFHS-2 results have clearly pointed out that the lack of knowledge of AIDS—its modes of transmission and ways to aviod infection—among women is a major challenge to efforts to avoid the spread of AIDS in India.

The Environment vis-à-vis the Vulnerability of Children to HIV/AIDS

Due to the invisibility of the people—adults and children—living with HIV/AIDS in India, the impact of the epidemic is also not visible. The invisibility of PLWHA is in part due to the current low levels of incidence in society as a whole in India and the social stigma usually associated with HIV, which results in those infected being reluctant to identify themselves as PLWHA.

A WHO study on individual and household responses in Mumbai found that some of the immediate impacts of infection included the withdrawal of children from school and early entry of children into the labour market (Bharat 1996). Illness or death of parents or guardians robs children of emotional and physical support and this situation is likely to be worse in poorer households. Before AIDS, one in 50 children in poor countries was an orphan; in some countries today, the rate is one in 10. Orphans, especially disadvantaged in terms of education due to the reduced ability of their families to pay school fees, are withdrawn from school to work for wages, help in family chores or care for ailing family members, as indicated in data from seven African countries, Haiti and Brazil (Mastro et al. 1998). Child malnutrition is one of the most severe and lasting consequences of death of the adult earner; it is a consequence of reduced household income, resulting in reduced food expenditure and a drop in food consumption. Very young orphans whose mothers are infected with HIV or die of AIDS have a higher mortality rate than other orphans because roughly one-third of them are themselves infected at or around the time of birth. The fear, discrimination, ignorance and social stigma associated with AIDS leaves affected children completely isolated.

Information on the number of infected children in India is not available, and, actually, the available data has not been disaggregated on the basis of age. In Maharashtra, a total of 215 mother-to-child-transmission (MTCT) cases of HIV and 44 of AIDS among children below the age of 14 years were reported during the period January–October 2000. Needless to say, this is a highly underestimated number. These are only those cases that go to public hospitals, and do not include individuals going to private hospitals or not seeking health services at all.

Although there are no accurate figures, NGOs estimate that there are at least 200,000 Nepali girls and women working in brothels in India. It is estimated that between 5,000 and 7,000 are annually trafficked into the industry (Haq 1997). More than 20 per cent of these girls are below 16 years of age. In June 1996, 124 commercially exploited girls in Mumbai were repatriated to Nepal; 60 per cent of these girls were HIV+ (Hannum 1997).

There is also very little information on the incidence of other STDs amongst children. One piece of information comes from a study at a private hospital in Delhi, which reported that 16 per cent of 362 STD cases were children under 14 years of age (private communication by Dr Jagannathan as reported in Ahmed 1998).

Such high incidence further emphasises the need for data to be collected on minors and then further disaggregated.

Certain cultural practices in India seem to make children, particularly girls, vulnerable to HIV/AIDS. One such practice is the system of the *devadasi*. A *devadasi* (literally meaning maidservant of God) is a young girl whose life is dedicated to the goddess Yellema, often when she is 4–5 years old. It is said that the girl has married God. Once a girl has been dedicated as a *devadasi*, she may never marry. One report suggests that about 15 per cent of all women in the sex industry in India have previously been *devadasis* (Narvesen 1989).

Street children, and again, more particularly girls, suffer a high incidence of sexual abuse, rape and victimisation. They are passive recipients of unsafe sexual practices that increase their risk of getting HIV/AIDS. It is reported that children on the streets, especially boys, are becoming sexually active between the ages of 7 and 9 years, and are at considerable risk of acquiring HIV/AIDS. Boys not only visit commercial sex workers but also practise male-to-male sex with boys and men (Ahmed 1998, CINI 1998). Children are less likely to use condoms than older men and women, and health care facilities are also often not geared to the needs of children. They aviod hospitals and even private practitioners for fear of being snubbed, and also because hospitals overawe them. Most of the boys prefer to go to the quacks or to the sex clinics which abound in the cities and which take advantage of all-round ignorance and myths about sex. In most cases, these children pay dearly for the wrong treatment they get when they go to quacks (Ahmed 1998).

Conclusion

In view of the evidence cited, which shows the great influence that environment has on the spread of HIV, it is obvious that without accounting for environmental factors, targeted interventions in India cannot achieve long-term behaviour change. While the focus of preventive programmes may continue to remain on addressing risky behaviour, a clear and realistic understanding of the context within which these behaviours occur would provide inputs into designing an effective strategy for behavioural change. It is also important to remember that it is not possible for a vertical programme to change the environment and that, therefore, an intersectoral approach to ensure an enabling environment would be prerequisite. The issue of safer sex will have to be addressed through a broader perspective and approach which is gender sensitive and encourages the participation of wider range of stakeholders. Some evidence to this nature is provided by sporadic NGO experiments (Verma et al. 1999). There is a need to seriously examine these experiments and evolve ways to upscale them. This will constitute the challenge in the coming years.

References/Further Reading

Ahmed, S., 1998. 'HIV/AIDS and Children: A South Asian Perspective'. Save the Children (UK) Office for South and Central Asia Region, Kathmandu.

Basu, A., D. Gupta and **G. Krishna,** 1995. 'The Household Impact of Adult Morbidity and Mortality: Some Implications of the Potential Epidemic of AIDS in India'. In *The Economics of HIV and AIDS*.

Bharat, S., 1996. *Facing the Challenge: Household and Community Response to HIV/AIDS in Mumbai*, India. Geneva: UNAIDS/TISS.

———, 1999. *HIV/AIDS Related Discrimination, Stigmatization and Denial in India: A Study in Mumbai and Bangalore*. UNAIDS, TISS.

CINI, 1998. A Report of the CINI-Asha Project in West Bengal.

Gangakhedkar, R.R., M.E. Bentley, A.D. Divekar, D. Gadkari, S.M. Mehendale, M.E. Shepherd, R.C. Bollinger, and **T.C. Quinn,** 1997. 'Spread of HIV Infection in Married Monogamous Women in India'. *JAMA*, 17 December, 278(23): 2090–92.

Hannum, J., 1997. *AIDS in Nepal: Communities Confronting an Emerging Epidemic*. New York: American Foundation for AIDS Research.

Haq, M.U., 1997. *Human Development in South Asia*. Karachi: Oxford University Press.

Hira, S., et al., 1998. 'HIV Infection in the Workforce and its Perceived Impact on Industry'. In P. Godwin (ed.), *The Looming Epidemic*, 139–49. New Delhi: Mosaic Books.

International Institute for Population Sciences, 2000. National Family Health Survey-2. Mumbai: International Institute for Population Sciences.

Lahiri, S., D. Balk and **K.B. Pathak,** 1995. 'Women in 13 States have Little Knowledge of AIDS'. National Family Health Survey Bulletin No. 2 (October), International Institute of Population Sciences, Mumbai, India and East West Center, Honolulu, USA.

Mane, P. and **S. Maitra,** 1992. *AIDS Prevention: The Socio-cultural Context in India*, Bombay: Tata Institute of Social Sciences.

Mastro, T.D., K.L. Zhang, S. Panda and **K.E. Nelson,** 1998. 'HIV Infection and AIDS in Asia'. In P.A. Pizzo and C.M. Wilfert (eds), *Paediatric Aids: The Challenge of HIV Infection in Infants, Children and Adolescents*, 3rd ed. Baltimore: Williams & Wilkins, pp. 47–63.

Mehendale, S., 1998. 'HIV Infection amongst Persons with High-Risk Behaviour in Pune City: Update on Findings from a Prospective Cohort Study'. *AIDS Research and Review*, 1: 2–9.

Mudur, G., 1998. 'Indian Supreme Court Rules that HIV Positive People Inform Spouses'. *BMJ*, 317: 1474.

National AIDS Control Organisation (NACO), 1997. *A Summary of the Findings of the High Risk Behavior Study from 18 Cities.* Ministry of Health and Family Welfare, Government of India.

————, 1999–2000. *Combating HIV/AIDS in India.* Ministry of Health and Family Welfare, Government of India.

Nag, M., 1996. *Sexual Behaviour and AIDS in India.* New Delhi: Vikas.

Narvesen, O., 1989. *The Sexual Exploitation of Children in Developing Countries.* Oslo: Redd Barna.

Panda, S., A. Chatterjee, S. Sarkar, K.N. Jalan, T. Maitra, S. Mukherjee, B. Mukherjee, B.C. Deb and **A.S. Abdul-Quader,** 1997. 'Injection Drug Use in Calcutta: A Potential Focus for an Explosive HIV Epidemic'. *Drug and Alcohol Review*, 16(1): 17–23.

Panda, S., A. Chatterjee, S.K. Bhattacharya, B. Manna, P.N. Singh, S. Sarkar, T.N. Naik, S. Chakrabarti and **R. Detels,** 2000. 'Transmission of HIV from Injecting Drug Users to their Wives in India'. *International Journal of STD and AIDS*, 11: 468–73.

Panda, S., L. Bijaya, S. Devi, E. Foley, A. Chatterjee, D. Banerjee, M.K. Saha, T.N. Naik and **S.K. Bhattacharya,** 2001. 'Interface of Drug and Sex in Imphal, Manipur'. *Nat Med J India*, 4: 209–11.

Pandav, C.S., K. Anand, B.R. Shamanna, S. Chowdhury and **L.M. Nath,** 1997. 'Economic Consequences of HIV/AIDS in India'. *Nat Med J India*, 10(1).

Pelto, P.J., A. Joshi and **R.K. Verma,** 2000. 'Development of Sexuality and Sexual Behaviour among Indian Males'. Paper presented in Asia Pacific Social Science and Medicine Conference, held at Kandy, Sri Lanka, 22–28 September.

Rao, A., M. Nag, K. Mishra and **A. Dey,** 1994. 'Sexual Behavior Pattern of Truck Drivers and their Helpers in Relation to Female Sex Workers'. *The India Journal of Social Work*, 55(4): 603–17.

Rangaiyan and **R.K. Verma,** 2001. *A Study of Sexual Behavior among College Students in Mumbai.* Mumbai: International Institute for Population Sciences.

Rodrigues, J.J., S.M. Mehendale, M.E. Shepherd, A.D. Divekar, R.R. Gangakhedkar, T.C. Quinn, R.S. Paranjape, A.R. Risbud, R.S. Brookmeyer, D.A. Gadkari, M.R. Gokhale, A.M. Rompalo, S.G. Deshpande, M.M. Khalandkar, N. Mawar, and **R.C. Bollinger,** 1995. 'Risk Factors for HIV Prevention in People Attending Clinics for sexually Transmitted Diseases in India'. *BMJ*, 311: 283–86.

Salunke, S.R., M. Shaukat, S.K. Hira and **M.R. Jagtap,** 1998. 'HIV/AIDS in India: A Country responds to a Challenge'. *AIDS*, 12 (Suppl. B): S27–S31.

Sharan, 1998. *Report on the Five-City Survey of IDUs.*

Shourie, L., 2000. 'HIV/AIDS Risk Behavior among IV Drug Users in Manipur and Its Correlate'. Unpulished Ph.D. thesis submitted to IIPS, Mumbai.

Singh, R., 1999. *HIV/AIDS, Workers and Labour Rights: A Study of Vulnerability of the Workers in Wazirpur Industrial Area, Delhi.* New Delhi: Centre for Education and Communication.

UNICEF/UNAIDS, December 1999. Call to Action for 'Children Left Behind by AIDS'.

Verma, R.K., A.A. Bhende and **P. Mane,** 1999. 'NGO Response to HIV/AIDS: A Focus on Women'. In Saroj Pachauri (ed.), *Implementing a Reproductive Health Agenda in India: The Beginning.* Population Council.

5

Community Responses to HIV/AIDS in Mumbai City

Shalini Bharat and *Peter Aggleton*

Introduction

Early on in the AIDS epidemic it became clear that HIV/AIDS is not just a biomedical problem but has sociocultural dimensions as well. Subsequently, there have been moves towards a more eco-logical understanding of vulnerability and responses to AIDS, which emphasise the role of households and communities. Although the importance of the extended family structure and kinship and clan systems in providing support has been demon-strated in several studies in Africa (Ankrah 1993, Barnett and Blaikie 1992, McGrath et al. 1993), few investigations have docu-mented and analysed the household and community context of AIDS in Asian countries. And yet, households and communities are expected to play important roles in mitigating the impact of the epidemic in some of the most resource-poor countries of Asia. This paper describes the community response to HIV/AIDS in a metropolis of India. It is based on a study (Bharat 1996) that was part of a larger multi-site research programme examining house-hold and community responses to HIV/AIDS in five developing countries—India, Mexico, Thailand, Tanzania and the Dominican Republic (WHO 1993). The broad objective of the study was to document household and community responses to HIV/AIDS as well as coping patterns, with a view to understanding the underlying sociocultural mechanisms determining these responses and developing household and community programmes and interventions to manage the epidemic. Descriptions of the household responses identified through the study can be found in two recent publications (Bharat and Aggleton 1999, Bharat et al. 1998).

The study was conducted in Brihan (Greater) Mumbai, the second-most populous city in India and its financial capital. Mumbai is located on the western coast in the state of Maharashtra, which has the highest recorded number of HIV and AIDS cases in India (NACO 1996). The city covers an area of nearly 600 sq. km. and the population is in the region of 9.9 million (Census of India 1991). Being a major commercial centre, the city has a large migrant population. Women are outnumbered by men to the ratio of 820 females per 1,000 males, compared to the state ratio of 936/1,000 and the national ratio of 929/1,000 (Census of India 1991). In-migration has made Mumbai an overcrowded, congested and polluted city, with nearly 40 per cent of the population estimated to be living in crowded and unhygienic conditions in nearly 570 slums.

Selection of Communities

For the purposes of this study, a community was understood as a neighbourhood or cluster of households within a defined geographical boundary. The selection of communities or neighbourhoods was guided by the presence of one or more households with HIV+ members recruited to participate in the study of household responses to HIV and AIDS. The selection of communities was carried out with the knowledge and cooperation of the positive people/household members, after they felt confident that the presence of project staff in their community would not threaten their identity.

Because a majority of the respondents came from low-income groups, the communities studied were impoverished. Two of them were slum communities (in the suburbs) and three were chawl[1] communities in Byculla, in the central part of the city. Access to all but one of the communities took place through youth clubs or community libraries, which are a characteristic feature of lower-class community life in Mumbai. In the Worli community, however, the point of entry was the household of a person living with HIV. Key informant interviews with doctors practising in each of these areas, youth club members, prominent members of the community iden- tified by others as 'social workers', and local political activists helped us build a socio-demographic profile of these communities. Eighteen focus group discussions (FGDs) were held with young (18–25 years) and older (30–45 years) community members of both genders to explore levels of awareness and understanding about HIV/AIDS, patterns of sexual behaviour, perceptions of the risk of HIV infection and ways of coping with the epidemic.

Establishing a Safe Environment for Information Seeking

It was realised that the presence of project staff in the communities could generate anxiety and suspicion about local cases of HIV. Project workers might be seen as health department workers trying to identify cases of HIV and AIDS, a parallel being drawn with the plague which had created panic in the city in October 1994. Staff members, therefore, explained their presence in more benign and general terms as seeking to understand health issues relevant to young people and adults in the community. Interviews and FGDs began by exploring general health problems in the community and only gradually turned to discussions of sexual bahaviour and issues related to HIV/AIDS. After some time in the community, however, it was possible to elicit a wide range of data about sexuality and HIV/AIDS. The discussions were conducted by a team consisting of a moderator and an observer matched for gender and language characteristics of the group. Discussions were tape recorded and later transcribed and translated into English. As far as possible, local terms and expressions were used to capture local meanings.

Description of the Communities

Slum 1 was a sprawling community located in the eastern suburb of Chembur along the eastern express highway. Slum 2 was located in the western suburb of Worli along the seashore and was much smaller in area and population than slum 1. In both these slums, the housing pattern consisted of rows of single or double storey, low-roofed brick houses separated by narrow paved lanes. Toilet blocks constructed on the fringes of the community were shared by the residents. The three chawls were located in central Mumbai. Chawls 1 and 2 were part of one complex and chawl 3 was part of another. These complexes were separated by a distance of approximately 3 km.

A room may have been occupied by a nuclear family or by an extended family consisting at times of 10–15 adult members and children. Sometimes a family may have taken in paying guests, thereby increasing the overcrowding. The common features of both chawl and slum communities were poor hygienic conditions, ill-ventilated rooms, lack of space, overcrowding and a concomitant lack of privacy. In particular, slum 1 and chawl 2 were extremely unhygienic, with overflowing drains, garbage littered all around and a larger number of people residing in each room. The slum population in general was poorer and lesser educated than the chawl population. A majority of the male residents of the chawls, with the exception of residents in chawl 2, worked as skilled low-ranked professionals (technicians, junior engineers) or in factories and private firms. The women were mainly housewives, but among those working, many were employed as teachers, nurses or community health workers. In chawl 2, the men were mainly employed as unskilled or semi-skilled workers and the women as domestic servants. In the slum population, the men were generally employed as low-skilled workers and sometimes as technicians, and the women as domestic servants or as maids in hospitals. A majority of the chawl residents (over 90 per cent) were Marathi or Konkani speaking. Slum 1 had a mixed population of natives and people from other states, whereas slum 2 consisted exclusively of migrant households living in the city.

The Findings

Contextualising HIV/AIDS

Initiation into sexual activities was reported as taking place at an age as low as 13–14 years for males, often in the company of older boys or under peer pressure to visit red-light districts. Fifty per cent, or, in one slum community, 80–90 per cent, of the males aged 14 years and above were said to visit commercial sex workers (CSWs). This behaviour was reported as particularly common among men with independent sources of income. School dropouts who joined the job market at a fairly young age also had the opportunity to spend at least a part of their income on themselves, and this included paying for various forms of entertainment or leisure activities, such as visiting sex workers, gambling, drinking and watching blue (pornographic) movies. Women tended to deny that their husbands visited red-light areas, or blamed themselves for it. As two of them put it,

> No man goes out if he has a wife at home. (Hirabai, Chembur slum)

> The doctor should not ask a woman suffering from boils [STDs] whether her husband visits sex workers … this way he puts a doubt in her mind. (Sheela, Byculla chawl 2)

But most women acknowledged that it was in men's nature to have sex outside a regular union, even when there was a 'good' wife at home. Married men often compared seeking paid sex to eating out in a restaurant despite food being available at home.

> Even if 'food' [at home] is good, you feel like eating out at a hotel. (Ganesh, Chembur slum)

> *Ghar ki murgi dhal barabar.* (The 'hen' at home is like ordinary grain.) (Majeed, Byculta chawl 2)

The lack of privacy at home due to overcrowding or the presence of children, though not explicitly cited as a reason, appeared to be a significant influencing factor in the sexual behaviour of couples and in the commercial sex-seeking behaviour of married men outside the household.[2] In some rooms, lofts had been constructed for the children or for younger couples, to provide some privacy. Many women (but few men) reported the presence of children or other adults in the same room as reasons for not having sex. Exhaustion from daily chores and tiredness from constant childbearing made some women lose interest in sex. Other women saw sex as an obligation on their part which had to be endured.

> Love-making is for husband's pleasure—it is a duty for his happiness. (Meena, Byculla chawl 2)
>
> It would be better to get rid of this headache [having sex]. (Kanta, Chembur slum)

But some women felt that if they continued to avoid having sex, their men would seek it out elsewhere. 'Men threaten that for four days you are saying "no" ... [and then they go to the sex workers],' as Sujataben of the Chembur slum said. In this kind of situation, sex workers provide an easy means of pleasure and relief to the men.

Not only men, but some housewives too were reported to engage in extramarital sex. The seduction of younger, unmarried men by older, married women was reported to be common by respondents in both the Byculla and Chembur communities, and was explained by factors as diverse as the husbands' alcoholism and habit of visiting sex workers, family violence and conflicts over finances. Individual interviews with unmarried, HIV+ men living in chawls also confirmed the involvement of some housewives in sexual relations with younger men.

The proliferation of liquor bars, screening of blue films in video parlours through the day, the easy availability of pornographic literature and movies, and the invasion of foreign television channels were reported as factors encouraging children to experiment with sex at an early age. Young men described the various methods that they as teenagers had devised for peeping into a neighbour's room or for witnessing adult sexual acts in the same room at night. These included removing tiles from roofs, boring holes in the walls or doors, pretending to be asleep, and so on.

Homosexual behaviour was cited in small numbers in all the communities. Various terms were used to refer to homosexuals—*goodh*, *chaukya* (a quarter less), *budhya*, etc., and the subject of homosexuality was discussed in a casual and light manner.

Socialisation for Reproductive Roles

Corroborating previous research (Bhende 1995), our study also showed that men and women lacked adequate knowledge about their bodies and about sex and sexuality. Boys and adult men shared misconceptions about physical and sexual weakness caused by semen loss through excessive masturbation, and thus justified their visits to CSWs to release 'heat'. Young boys expressed the need for more scientific information on physical and sexual development. Several cheaply priced magazines in English, Hindi and the vernacular languages, such as *Dhadakti Jawani* (pulsating youth) were mentioned as sources of both vicarious pleasure and information on sex.

FGDs conducted with unmarried adolescent girls and recently married young women revealed the inadequate preparation with which women crossed the threshold of sexual activity, marriage and motherhood. Their experiences with menstruation and the manner in which they had been oriented to this critical phase that bore significance for their reproductive roles made the culture of silence strikingly clear. The following quotes reflect the girls' lack of preparation, their sense of 'shyness' and 'shame' connected with their emerging sexuality and polluting bodies, and the mothers' fears about their daughters' sexual vulnerability.

> No, mother had not told me anything about it [menstrual period]. (Lata, Byculla chawl 1)

> [When I first saw blood] I thought I had hurt myself. (Sunita, Byculla chawl 3)

> I thought that I had contracted some horrible disease, that I was dying. (Pinky, Chembur slum)

> I was told I was a grown up girl now. I should not roam around with boys ... I should behave with dignity lest I ruin my family's izzat [honour]. (Meena, Byculla chawl 3)

> I felt wretched and ashamed ... what a life for we womenfolk. Absolutely third rate! (Rani, Byculla chawl 1)

Underlying this culture of silence are the social norms that expect 'good' girls to be innocent about sex and the reproductive function of their bodies, thereby curbing any curiosity, and even genuine need for help regarding problems, associated with sex and reproduction. The women at first generally denied any sexual health problems and STDs. It was only after some amount of probing that many married women mentioned problems such as foul-smelling white discharge, vaginal itching and boils, burning sensation while urinating, delayed or irregular menstruation and pain in the lower back. Seeking medical care for these problems was difficult, they said; first, on account of the high fee charged by the local doctors and second, because medical treatment provided only temporary relief each time, not a cure. They blamed the doctors for wrong diagnoses and for providing incomplete treatment.

Knowledge and Awareness of HIV/AIDS

AIDS had no specific name in the community. It was commonly recognised as a dreadful (*bhayanak*), incurable (*illaj nahin hai*) and dirty disease (*gandi bimari*) contracted by having sexual relations 'outside', going to 'those bad women' (*woh gandi auratein*) and engaging in multipartner sex. The 'sex connection' in AIDS was thus widely shared across age groups and genders. AIDS was usually described as a disease that had come from abroad and was seen as linked to some 'defect' or 'mistake' in the blood. In terms of severity and extent of infection, people tended to draw parallels with tuberculosis, a disease which is rampant in these same settings. Accordingly, they talked of stages of infection ('first stage' or 'last stage') and the extent of the damage ('little' or 'too much'). They also tended to quantify the infection in much the same way as is done with tuberculosis (small or large patch on the lungs), which also provides evidence of the chances of getting cured. Not many people had heard about HIV, and those who had could not clearly distinguish between HIV and AIDS. Very few people knew that HIV is the name of the micro-organism (*jeevanu*) that causes AIDS.[3] About 70 per cent of the interviewees (more men than women) knew about modes of infection other than sex, such as through infected blood and from a pregnant woman to the foetus. When asked about who and what caused the infection, people uniformly said that prostitutes were its source. 'Prostitutes are the agents...,' said Mahesh of the Chembur slum, and 'Prostitutes are the spreading medium...,' claimed Namdev of Byculla chawl 2.

But some people (both men and women) perceived women in general, including housewives, as the source of the infection.

> Housewives can also give ... some housewives have relations with ten–ten men.... (Namdev, Byculla chawl 2)
>
> Some women are also bad ... not only men.... (Kishore, Byculla chawl 2)

Some men considered middle-aged women to be particularly responsible.

> Women aged 32–39 years have double sexual energy, so they look for younger/older men other than their husbands.... (Sanjeev, Byculla chawl 1)

While men generally made little reference to the fact that they too could infect their sexual partners, the women seemed more informed about this.

> Men who visit prostitutes give it to the poor wife.... (Meena, Byculla chawl 1)

> Men spend time with bar girls ... and they have AIDS ... and they give it to the men, who come home [with the infection].... (Sumitra Bai, Byculla chawl 2)

Discussion about who could become infected showed that people participating in high-risk behaviour were considered more likely to contract the infection.

> Men who go 'out', homosexuals, beer bar girls, 'bad women' and 'ones who step aside [from the right path]....' (18–25-year-old males, Byculla chawl 1)

There was also a fatalistic attitude about AIDS. As one focus group member put it, 'One who is fated to get, will get it, others won't get....' Some men held the view that AIDS spreads faster among men and that it is not so much of a problem among women.

> ... it does not spread so easily among women, it stays like that only ... like you said the prostitute is like an agent ... she remains as an agent, she does not have trouble, but ... because of her, those who go to her get the trouble.... (Vikas, Byculla chawl 3)

Similarly, although people said that unsterilised and re-used needles/syringes and infected blood can cause AIDS, they rarely mentioned injecting drug users (IDUs), blood donors or the recipients of blood products, such as haemophiliacs and pregnant women, as among those likely to become infected. In other words, AIDS was perceived mainly in the context of heterosexual transmission and with reference to paid-for sex and/or casual and multi-partner sex—a view that largely explains the society's moralistic and judgemental attitudes towards people living with HIV/AIDS (PLWHA).

Misconceptions About HIV/AIDS

Some basic facts about the causes of HIV/AIDS were correctly known to the majority of the respondents, but there were doubts and misconceptions in several areas. Although a majority of the interviewees said that AIDS was not spread by physical touch, hugging, kissing, eating together, shaking hands or by sharing clothes, some held grave misconceptions.

> It may spread through mosquito bites and flies.... (Dileep, Byculla chawl 3)

> If one in the family has, everybody can get it.... (Kishore, Byculla chawl 2)

> Barber's blade can also give the infection if he does not change it.... (Sanjeev, Byculla chawl 1)

> Micro-organisms [of AIDS] fall through air.... (Santosh, Chembur slum)

> A tiny dot of blood can also infect.... (Namdev, Byculla chawl 2)

> Upon contact with our body it [the virus] can immediately cause AIDS.... (Sumitra Bai, Byculla chawl 2)

> Its virus can spread by talking to the infected person.... (Krupashankar, Byculla chawl 3)

> Only when a man dies, the [AIDS] virus can spread, virus comes out when a man dies.... (Mahesh, Chembur slum)

> If a man has relations with wife during menstruation, he can get AIDS.... (Prakash, Byculla chawl 2)

Fear of urinals as possible sources of infection was particularly prevalent among a group of older married men.

> The gases from the urinals ... when our urine falls on others' urine ... the gases that flow out can cause the disease. In the areas where prostitution goes on, the urinals are very dirty. Insecticides should be sprayed.... (Saleem, Chembur slum)

Advertisements on television, posters in municipal hospitals and trains, and newspaper reports were cited as common sources of information. But, sometimes, these were sources of confusion too. For instance, one frequently cited advertisement features a popular Hindi film star, Shabana Azmi, hugging a child as she talks about modes of transmission. The visual of a child as a patient in a hospital ward which journalists were hesistant to enter, gave some women the impression that only children get AIDS.

> Does it mean that only children get AIDS? Shabana hugs a small child in the hospital so.... (Surekha, Byculla chawl 1)

One community health worker described her own experience in this respect.

> At our place [of residence] it is generally understood that this disease happens only to small children ... now where do small children go to get this disease? I tried to explain to those women but [somebody's] mother-in-law argued so much with me because in the advertisement they show a pregnant woman and they show Shabana hugging a child ... that is all those women understand. Actually the advertisement shows the back [of a man] with arms [embracing him] but ... what will these women understand ... what they hear ... they see a 'big' stomach and this small girl with HIV.... How to make this mother-in-law understand? She asked me how do you know... [now] this is also a problem. Finally, what to tell such people? (Tarabai, local health worker at Byculla)

A poster in a municipal hospital was similarly misinterpreted thus.

> The poster says you must not come very close to a woman when talking, and you need to keep a distance from her mouth.... (Savitri, Byculla chawl 3)

Misconceptions and confusions also existed due to peoples' observations of how medical professionals in hospitals responded to PLWHA and the instructions given to family members of patients who were suspected of having HIV.

> Advertisements say that it is not a contagious disease then why do doctors and nurses not touch them.... (Balram, Byculla chawl 3)

> If it is not a contagious disease then why was ... [somebody's] wife asked to wear gloves and mask when entering his room? (Malanbai, Byculla chawl 1]

Symptoms of AIDS

Most respondents said they had not seen a person with AIDS and, therefore, they could not say anything about its symptoms. But they associated certain physical manifestations with cases of AIDS. A person with AIDS was generally described as someone who lost her/his resistance and power, grew weak and thin, and then:

> His bones become powdery and useless like in paralysis. AIDS viruses go into the marrow of the bones and grow there, so they become weak.... (Sanjeev, Byculla chawl 1)
>
> Body turns black.... (Meena, Byculla chawl 1)
>
> The blood solidifies.... (Vikas, Byculla chawl 3)
>
> Instead of urine they pass red water and develop red and yellow spots on eyes, and their body turns yellow.... (Balram, Byculla chawl 3)

It was commonly believed that AIDS is a 'thinning' disease in which the body loses its power of resistance and the person becomes weak and skeleton-like.

Experiencing AIDS in the Community

In all the communities except the Worli slum, people at first denied the presence of AIDS in their midst. During discussions, however, several participants identified individuals who they suspected of having or having had AIDS for reasons including unexplained long-term illness, swift death, and physical symptoms such as the body turning black. Additionally, specific precautions which had been recommended by doctors and the manner of disposing dead bodies were further sources of evidence used to make putative AIDS diagnoses. Normally, most AIDS cases were described as tuberculosis cases by family members. But at the level of community perceptions, tuberculosis was not believed to be a killer disease if timely treatment was provided. Therefore, any illness that did not respond to treatment was suspected of being AIDS.

> Tuberculosis gets cured these days, then what illness is this that does not get cured, I suppose it was AIDS.... (Sanjeev, Byculla chawl 1)

People also cited occasions when family members had been advised to wear gloves and a mask when taking care of an ill person, giving rise to the speculation that the patient was probably suffering from AIDS. Suicide by some ill members of the communities also gave rise to suspicions that they had been people with AIDS who had been afraid of the social consequences of the disease for them and their families. If these persons had happened to belong to high-risk groups, the suspicion of AIDS was even stronger.

In the Chembur slum, the death of a bar girl in 1994 was widely attributed to AIDS and led to a great deal of fear, especially among some boys known to have been friendly with her. They expressed the need to be tested for HIV.

> An 18-year-old bar girl burned herself to death ... she was an AIDS patient.... (Mahesh, Chembur slum)

> The person who died was a bar girl, probably she died of AIDS.... (Santosh, Chembur slum)

In the Byculla area, the disposal of a few dead bodies from hospitals in black plastic bags tied at the mouth, with strict instructions to family members not to open the bags, had led to a lot of speculation among community members as to the nature of the dead persons' illness and the cause of the deaths. The people in one chawl described the events.

> When the dead body arrived it was wrapped in a black plastic bag. We were all very curious ... we had never seen a dead body being brought in this way. The family members did not even open the bag to show the face ... and they quickly took it away ... we don't know the reason, but it looked strange. (Prakash, Byculla chawl 2)

In the Worli slum, the family members of a deceased person with AIDS described the manner in which they were handed the body.

> We were given the body in a plastic bag and the hospital people said that you should not open the bag because the AIDS germs will fly out and harm you. So, if you open you will do so at your risk. We are not to be blamed then. So, we didn't think of bringing the body home because anyway we could not have performed the last rites. (Kanamma, Worli slum)

Overall, the communities studied were experiencing the epidemic in an atmosphere of suspicion and anxiety, one fuelled by local understandings and images of AIDS.

Perception of Risk of Infection in the Community

Opinion was divided as to whether there was risk of infection in the communities studied. Despite acknowledging the practice of multipartner sex among the male members of their communities, many people (both women and men) said that there was no possibility of AIDS being in their communities because so far they had not seen any cases of AIDS in their neighbourhood. This non-visibility of confirmed cases made people feel less vulnerable to infection. Comparatively better educated married men from one chawl believed that:

> Those who are educated have television and newspapers for information and therefore can take precautions ... it is the illiterate people living in the slums who lack such sources of information and need to be told.... (Narayan, Byculla chawl 3)

The dominant attitude here was that:

> We have not seen AIDS patient because it has not spread among the educated middle class.... (Balram, Byculla chawl 3)

> We don't go to prostitutes, so we won't get AIDS.... (Narayan, Byculla chawl 3)

In short, AIDS was seen as a problem of the lesser educated and of those who visited sex workers. In one of the slums, however, a group of married men in the late 1930s opined that:

> Men like us who have sexual relations with our wife any number of time will not get AIDS. (Sambhoji, Worli slum)

The possibility of becoming infected through means other than the sexual route was not envisaged. Most people felt that younger, college-going boys were more likely to be at risk of infection because of their more permissive sexual behaviour. Younger men, for their part, also seemed to perceive in themselves a greater vulnerability to AIDS. During their fieldwork, the organisers of an AIDS awareness camp in one chawl reported that fewer younger men had attended the programmes, possibly because they had feared that their presence would be nagatively construed. But the FGDs in the Chembur slum caused many young men to reflect on their behaviour, and some subsequently contacted the project staff for the addresses of HIV testing centres, AIDS counselling centres and for literature on AIDS. They also requested the project staff to organise extra AIDS awareness sessions because they identified the younger men of their community as especially vulnerable to infection in view of their unsafe sexual behaviour.

Housewives, however, tended to see themselves as much less vulnerable. 'What AIDS! ... are we those kinds of women ... as if we will get it [AIDS]...' (Surekha, Byculla chawl 1). Generally, it was sex workers who were seen as most vulnerable, not women who stayed at home. This attitude was reinforced by health workers too. At an AIDS awareness camp for women, for example, Kumud, a community health worker at Byculla, said to the participants: 'We are all family women here ... so there is no question of sexual relations outside....' The discussion then moved on to high-risk behaviour groups.

Prevention of AIDS

Within the context of heterosexual transmission, AIDS prevention was largely understood only in relation to sex workers.

> Men should not visit sex workers ... and if they do, they should use Nirodh [brand name of a condom]. (Dileep, Byculla chawl 3)

Some men considered it the sex workers' responsibility to ensure that men used condoms.

> The prostitute should be told that see if you are in this job ... and if you want to live your life, then you must do all this [ask men to use condoms] ... if you do then your life will increase and the other person's life also. (Namdev, Byculla chawl 2)

In addition, condoms were seen as suitable for use only when having sex outside the home, ignoring the possibility of HIV transmission from men to their wives and other regular sex partners. Dileep from Byculla chawl 3 said, 'At home there is no need to use Nirodh ... the wife is pure'.

Advertisements advising the use of condoms, even at home, were dismissed as applicable only to upper-income groups where it was believed that wives may be unfaithful to their husbands.

Men from the lower middle class, chawl 3 especially, did not consider the use of condoms proper for them. Women's attitudes towards the condom were linked to more general beliefs about sex. 'It is for his pleasure that he comes to us for sex, so he should wear it ... ,' said Sujataben, Chembur slum.

Some women felt that it was important for their own safety that condoms were used, but were unsure about how to insist upon their usage with their husbands. In this connection they drew a distinction between sensible, or responsible, and irresponsible men. 'If the man is sensible he will use Nirodh ... ,' Sujataben said.

Besides condoms, a very small number of people mentioned the use of disposable, needles, and the testing of blood before blood transfusion as strategies for AIDS prevention.

Community Responses to People Living with HIV/AIDS

The communities studied have generally responded to HIV/AIDS as an epidemic, and not referred to individual people living with HIV/AIDS because there were no confirmed or self-disclosed cases of AIDS in the selected communities, with the exception of the Worli slum. With a view to better understanding community response to persons with AIDS, therefore, two hypothetical situations were presented in discussions with two groups, one each of men and women, in chawl 2. One situation invloved a young widow with HIV and her two young children who were driven out of her in-laws' house. What, we asked, would be the community's response if this widow was living in their neighbourhood? People said that they would provide financial help and ask the widow to see a doctor. They said that they would arrange for her children to be looked after in an institution where support would be available from social workers. But they were not sure that they could intervene in the household's internal matters so as to impress upon the in-laws the need to take care of the woman. Moreover, they said that their own family members might not like the idea of them interfering in other people's affairs.

The other hypothetical situation involved the owner of a tea stall in their community which they had been patronising for a long time. If this tea stall owner were to test HIV+, we asked, would they continue to buy tea from his stall. The respondents were near unanimous in saying that they would ask the owner to leave the tea business and seek treatment, and that they would not drink tea from his stall. 'We know that we will not catch infection like this, but yet in our mind we think we can get. Then why test it [why take a chance],' said Kanta of Byculla chawl 2.

Discussing hypothetical situations is obviously not the ideal way of highlighting all the issues linked to a sensitive subject such as AIDS. More direct experiences reported as having taken place in the Worli slum provided us an opportunity to understand community responses to people with HIV/AIDS from a closer angle. There were four confirmed cases of HIV/AIDS (2 men and 2 women) within this community at the time of our visit, but the other members were demanding the expulsion of only one particular person from the community and advising that he be moved to a hospital. This person was an HIV+ man suffering from diarrhoea, skin infections and tuberculosis. He was very thin and could barely walk. His skin had turned very dark and was beginning to peel off. The other three community members who were infected were not being discriminated against. We explored why this was the case in the focus group discussions with members of the community. They revealed that they perceived the person whose expulsion was being demanded as a threat to their health.

> He defecates and urinates in the open space close to our houses, where our children play. The germs from his urine can rise up. He spits everywhere and we feel he could pass on the infection. He looks scary too ... children are afraid to see him at night. We are saying that he should not be kept at home, but in the hospital. (Chandran, Worli slum)

When asked why the three other cases were not being discriminated against, members of the community said:

> The other three people are confined to their houses and carry on with their household work ... they have no external symptoms and they behave responsibly. That is, they do not spit, etc. ... then why should we say anything to them.... (Chandran, Worli slum)

The wife of the person whom the community did not want in their midst was naturally very upset and angry, and she was actually the one to reveal the AIDS status of the other three people in public. Until then, no one in the community had understood that these three people also had AIDS. The wife felt that she and her husband were being discriminated against because they were poorer and because there was nobody to speak out on their behalf.

Conclusion

Although Mumbai is called the AIDS capital of India, the HIV epidemic in the city is in many ways still invisible. What this means is that, for the local people, familiarity with the epidemic comes mainly through media advertisements and slogans. Because people with HIV and AIDS and their households remain largely hidden, the epidemic has still to take a human face. However, people's curiosity and anxiety about unexplained illnesses, unusual medical advice, and the return of the bodies of a few deceased people in sealed black plastic bags is giving rise to suspicions about the possibility of AIDS in their midst. This has also made it easier to speculate about who might be at risk. Bar girls, sex workers and younger men who frequent brothels and bars remain among those assumed to be especially vulnerable. In order to give a human face to the epidemic and to normalise it, awareness programmes must try to personalise HIV/AIDS. Positive people, willing to be open about their status (even if selectively, that is, only with some, and not all, people) can spearhead community awareness programmes. However, these people should be backed by strong care and counselling programmes.

One of the main problems facing PLWHA in coming out in public is their apprehension of being isolated, rejected and stigmatised in their neighbourhoods, social circles and among relatives. Consequently, community resources, such as, peer group support, counselling from older members, neighbourly concern and care, remain untapped. Communities, on the other hand, are apprehensive and suspicious about 'AIDS-like cases,' and need to understand that their responses reflect anxieties and fears about the unknown. But the findings of this study suggest that community responses are not always negative. When a person is largely asymptomatic and not seen as posing a threat to others, both acceptance and tolerance have been shown towards the person.

This suggests that if households are helped to manage members who are sick as a result of AIDS such that they are not perceived as a threat to other's health, communities can be expected to respond in a more responsible and positive manner.

The findings reaffirm the poor knowledge base of the communities with respect to HIV/AIDS. Because misconceptions and doubts remain, there is an urgent need for creating AIDS knowledge and awareness in communities. But young people and women feel threatened when seen attending AIDS-related programmes. Therefore, for creating acceptance among people, these programmes should be included in ongoing health programmes such as, reproductive health and family life education.

Public information campaigns and media advertisements appear to have been both a source of information and confusion. This is so because some of the existing education and awareness programmes are loaded with slogans and statements that are not clear-cut in their message and that fail to highlight the link between HIV/AIDS and individual's own risk behaviour. Worse, there is no way people can correct their misconceptions or seek clarification because community-level efforts for creating awareness are sorely lacking. There is, thus, a need to develop innovative and thoughtful education programmes that will involve participation from people and, above all, make them seriously think about their vulnerability and the need to adopt preventive and protective methods. Negative campaigning and fear-inducing messages ('AIDS means death') must be given up for messages that encourage responsible behaviour. The visibility of available sources of information, education, care and counselling among community members also needs to be enhanced. It is very important that people know where to go for HIV testing, counselling, support and information.

Despite self-acknowledged high levels of risk behaviour, assessments of personal risks of infection were generally poor. A disturbing finding was that sex workers and, in some communities, housewives too, were considered to be the main vectors of HIV infection. Condom usage was seen as appropriate largely in the context of sex outside the home and not between spouses. A healthy and encouraging finding, however, was the higher levels of awareness and concern generated among the younger men following focus group discussions. This was reflected in their health seeking behaviour and their desire to have more knowledge and information about HIV/AIDS.

At this stage of the epidemic in Mumbai, when some communities are beginning to become curious and suspicious about AIDS and are creating their own images of the epidemic, and when younger men in particular are expressing a need for more information, innovative and credible AIDS education and prevention programmes are much needed. 'Strike while the iron is hot' is the phrase which most aptly describes the prevention strategy needed in the communities studied in Mumbai.

Notes

1. Chawls are 5–6 storeys-high single-room tenement buildings with common passageways and shared toilet(s) on each floor. Rooms measure approximately 10 × 15 feet and are used for both living and cooking purposes, and a corner of the room is used as a wash area (*mori*).
2. Overcrowding is a common feature of slum and chawl living. Two or three couples with young children and other adults such as parent(s) in many cases stay in one single room.
3. During discussions, people referred to the epidemic mainly as AIDS. Hence, this word is used throughout this chapter.

References/Further Reading

Ankrah, E.M., 1993. 'The Impact of HIV/AIDS on the Family and other Significant Relationships: The African Clan Revisited'. *AIDS Care*, 5, 5–22.

Barnett, T. and P. Blaikie, 1992. *AIDS in Africa: Its Present and Future Impact*. London: Belhaven Press.

Bharat, S., 1996. *Facing the Challenge: Household and Community Responses to HIV/AIDS in Mumbai, India*. Mumbai: TISS (GPA/WHO, Geneva).

Bharat, S. and P. Aggleton, 1999. 'Facing the challenge: Household Responses to AIDS in Mumbai, India'. *AIDS Care*, 11:1, 31–44.

Bharat, S., A. Singhanetra-Renard and P. Aggleton, 1998. 'Household and Community Responses to HIV/AIDS in Asia: The Case of Thailand and Asia'. *AIDS*, 12 (Supplement B): S117–S122.

Bhende, A., 1995. *Evolving a Model for AIDS Prevention Education among Underprivileged Adolescent Girls in Urban India* (Women and AIDS Program Research Report Series). Washington, D.C.: International Center for Research on Women.

Census of India, 1991. Maharashtra Provision Population Totals, Series 14, Paper I, Mumbai.

McGrath, J.W., W. Ankrah, D.A. Schumann, S. Nkumbi and **M. Lubega,** 1993. 'AIDS in the Urban Family: Its Impact in Kampala, Uganda'. *AIDS Care*, 5: 55–70.

National AIDS Control Organisation (NACO), 1996. Country Scenario: An Update. New Delhi: Ministry of Health and Family Welfare, Government of India.

World Health Organization, 1993. *Household and Community Responses to HIV/AIDS: A General Research Protocol.* Geneva: World Health Organization, Global Programme on AIDS, Social and Behavioural Studies Support Unit.

6

Interventions among Men Who Have Sex with Men

K. Pradeep

Introduction

Since 1986, when the first HIV+ female sex worker was identified in Tamil Nadu, it has been generally believed in India that AIDS is heterosexually transmitted and that its spread in India will follow the African scenario (ICMR 1992). This idea is strengthened by the widespread belief that homosexuality does not exist in India and on the available epidemiological data.[1] In India, homo-sexuality as a concept is linked with the United States of America and other countries in the Western hemisphere.

In the beginning of the 1990s, different opinions about homo-sexuality in India were voiced by groups such as Bombay Dost. The mere existence of this organisation proved that there was something other than heterosexuality in India as well. Bombay Dost had also discretely made it known they feared their com-munity to be at high risk for HIV infection. In 1993, a study con-ducted in Mumbai (then Bombay) revealed that 'the homosexual transmission of HIV infection is not uncommon in a metropolitan city like Bombay' (Nandi et al. 1994). While there was a growing acceptance that homosexuality behaviour was prevalent in India, it was still believed to be restricted to major cities and, particularly, Mumbai (Devi 1997, Arvind 1991, Row Kavi 1991).

While more recently a number of gay and lesbian groups have emerged throughout the country,[2] most so-called homosexuals are not identifiable and are quite blended into society (the male world) at large. Men who have a feminine strain in their gender identity or who have an exclusive preference for the same sex are largely underground and not out in the open.

Very few men in India openly express an identity based on their sexual preference and call themselves 'gay'. This does not mean there are not many homosexuals, nor that homosexual activity is not highly prevalent; only that this activity is not visible. It is in most cases not linked with a lifestyle and a public identity. Legal, cultural, social and religious sanctions increase the invisibility of homosexual roles and identities (McKenna 1996).

The uncritical use of Western categories of sexuality in discussing men who have sex with men (MSM) in the Indian context adds to the confusion over identities. Many societies do not even have a term for homosexual, reflecting the fact that 'homosexual' and 'heterosexual' are terms coined only in the last century in Europe (Tan 1994).

In the traditional Indian sexual culture there exists the specific construction of a third gender (not man, not woman), called Hijra in the north and Ali in the south. Hijra/Ali comes close to the Western transsexual (men who identify as women and have the desire for a sex change). In traditional Indian society, Hijra/Ali played a religious role, but in more recent times this function has eroded. More and more Hijras and Alis resort to prostitution to make a living.

Due to the strict segregation of female and male, many Indian men do not relate socially with women. For the Indian male the female world is strange and largely not understood. Even in marriage, social interaction between husband and wife is limited. The social roles of husband and wife are clearly defined and separated. Often, the contact between man and woman within marriage is only sexual. On the other hand, as if as a compensation, there is strong homosocial bonding. Men relate socially with other men. Though homosocial and homosexual should not be mixed up, the divide between social and sexual in male–male relations is fluid and not very sharp.

Hijra and Ali, effeminate men, androgynous boys with smooth and fair skin and men who have a feminine appearance are often more easily approachable for masculine men who have not learned to socially relate with women. It may be for this reason that many Indian men have sex with 'in between' men. It is easy for them to relate with them and they are sexually attractive enough because they are a bit feminine. As in other fields of culture, illusion and fantasy perhaps fill the gaps. The 'in between' boys and men and the third gender bridge the abyss between the male and female worlds. This is the most striking difference between Western and Indian sexual cultures. The Indian system of three genders, with unique linkages, versus a disciplined Western system of two genders in which those who do not fit in have been set apart, given rights and respect, but sexually unlinked and isolated.

This paper attempts to provide a background on MSM in India and looks at the sociocultural realities that determine sexual construction. It also explores in detail the interventions for HIV/AIDS prevention amongst MSM and the Ali community in Chennai while providing an overview of similar attempts in other parts of the country. The inclusion of Ali in the MSM category is debatable. They are indeed separate and culturally a third gender in the Indian context but, for want of space, are part of this chapter.

Ethnography of Men Who Have Sex with Men in Chennai

Through support from the WHO's Global Programme on AIDS (GPA), a number of situational assessments were undertaken in Chennai, Tamil Nadu, in 1992 and 1993. The objective of these assessments was to determine the need for targeted HIV/AIDS prevention in particular settings and, once that was done, to provide descriptive information from which intervention strategies could be developed. One such assessment was conducted over a six-month period in 1993 on the occurrence of male homosexual contacts in diverse contexts, including that of male prostitutes (NACP et al. 1993).

Using ethnographic methods the assessment of homosexual contacts identified numerous cruising areas, or public sex environments

(PSEs), such as parks and beach-side promenades, which are regularly visited by men who have sex with men. In addition to describing the characteristics of those frequenting PSEs, the assessment found that unprotected penetrative sex was common among men with multiple sexual partners. In addition, some MSM had casual or regular female sex partners, with the latter usually being unaware of their partners' homosexual contacts.[3] Such practices occur in the broader context of limited awareness of HIV/AIDS.

In Chennai, men involved in same-sex contacts do not necessarily identify as homosexual. The understanding of homosexuality in India, like in many other societies,[4] draws on the distinction between those who prefer the 'active' as opposed to the 'passive' role in sex.

While HIV prevalence among MSM is thought to be less than that among female sex workers, the number of infections is increasing among all populations involved in multi-partner sexual contacts (John et al. 1993). Underreporting of homosexual contacts is also a significant factor in this context (Orton 1995).

Results of the Ethnography in Chennai

Situational assessment and outreach encounters since early 1994 provide the estimate that between 5,000 and 6,000 persons are regularly involved in homosexual contacts at PSEs in Chennai.[5] The PSEs are spread throughout the city and could be parks, beaches, along deserted rail tracks, theatres, etc. Over 70 such cruising points were mapped in the city, with 10 of them getting over 150 MSM cruising on a daily basis. The number of cruising MSM peaks during the weekends, with some of these cruising points getting between 300 and 400 MSM on Saturdays and Sundays.

A number of deaths from AIDS in the Ali community and public disclosure by homosexual men of their seropositivity has increased concern about the risk of HIV infections in these two populations. Regardless of current prevalence rates, unprotected penetrative sex with multiple partners was found to be widespread, perception of STD and HIV risks were low and condom usage largely non-existent. The ethnographic study also revealed that many did not know that unprotected homosexual contact could lead to HIV infection.

Targeted intervention to reduce the considerable risks of infection among MSM and Alis was deemed essential in this context. The specific objectives of the intervention were

- to promote condom use in all penetrative sexual intercourse
- to encourage a shift towards less risky sexual practices
- to provide prevention education on HIV/AIDS and STDs
- to facilitate greater access to STD care and health care in general.

In the particular case of the Ali community, because of their marginal socio-economic and health status, AIDS prevention efforts have been addressed within broader socio-economic and health concerns.

The intervention strategies designed to meet these objectives were determined to a great extent by the existence of specific entry points to this risk setting. The two most important entry points are PSEs and socio-sexual networks among MSM. Interaction between MSM is defined by friendship ties or common sexual interests, while a community structure exists for transsexuals which makes possible collective action.

In the case of men who cruise the PSEs, person-to-person outreach encounters provided an opportunity for AIDS education. For transsexuals, two strategies were initiated—the first was to use a core group of peer educators selected from among the prominent figures, or *gurus,* of the community to promote safer sex practices, and the second was to address some of the difficulties characteristic of their living conditions. Examples of the latter include assistance in putting forward demands to public housing authorities, reducing discriminatory treatment on the part of health workers and, in a few cases, providing opportunities for vocational training.

Among MSM, the original protocol separates out those involved in prostitution as 'commercial boys' from those searching for non-paying sexual partners. In practice, however, this distinction is difficult to maintain given that the two take place in the same population and that a person may sometimes be actively searching for money in exchange for sex while at other times he is seeking a non-paying sexual partner. However, an effort was made to include a core group of peer educators who are predominantly involved in prostitution.

Underlying the choice of intervention strategies is the diffusion model of HIV/AIDS related prevention messages and the introduction of condom use where previously it did not exist. The establishment of safer sex practices was initially encouraged among persons the project was in contact with, who, in turn, served to diffuse prevention messages through peer contacts to the population concerned. AIDS education is also supported by the establishment of condom distribution, facilitated access to STD or other health services and the organisation of social activities specific to this population (such as, participation in the annual festival for transsexuals in India).

MSM do not necessarily self-identify as gay or homosexual. To a certain extent, outside the PSEs, they may not perceive themselves as having a sexual identity distinct from that of other men. For most MSM, marriage remains a likely or inevitable option. In a few cases, marriage is encouraged precisely because the family suspects or knows of the sexual orientation of the son.

Those visiting PSEs usually change partners frequently and have diverse sexual practices which include anal and oral sex. However, the frequency of sexual practices varies at different PSEs. While the majority of sexual contacts do not involve the exchange of money, there are networks of young men or commercial boys who do engage in sex work. Some engage in sex work on an occasional basis, while others are part of a more professional network who have brokers to contact clients. Commercial boys occupy specific turf at PSEs and usually operate in the late hours of the night.

Three main categories were identified among those involved in homosexual contact at the PSEs.

Danga is similar to rani (in Hindi) and queen (in English). It is a term used to classify men with a very strong feminine strain in their gender identity. Sexually, *dangas* prefer to be receptive partners in anal intercourse and to be the performers of fellatio. They often walk and talk like women, especially when out cruising. When in a group, they jokingly refer to each other as sisters and talk in terms of 'she' when referring to other *dangas*.

Panthi, or butch, refers to men with a masculine identity and a predominant sexual orientation towards women. *Panthi* is a category used by *dangas* to indicate that a man is a real man, which in their view means he should always be the inserter in anal intercourse and undergo fellatio. *Panthis* who sell oral sex, for instance, are no longer seen as real *panthis*.

Double Decker is used by Alis and *dangas* to mark men who like sex with other men. The prime distinction between double decker and *panthi* is that the former also like the male sexual organ. They both receive and perform fellatio. They are both receptive and inserting partners in anal intercourse. In case they look masculine they are also liked by Alis for sex. For most die-hard *dangas* the mere fact that a man performs fellatio on another man disqualifies him as a potential sexual, and even social, partner. Remarkably, this is not the case for Alis, many of whom enjoy double deckers.

While this classification is not obvious to those external to the subculture, it is used by MSM themselves to identify potential partners.

Ali is the traditional Tamil construction of a third gender. Alis are considered neither men nor women. They have very strong community ties and live in groups, often on the outskirts of the cities. While in the north they play a religious role in marriage and birth rituals, in modern Tamil society their status is rapidly deteriorating. It is estimated that some 300 Alis sell sex in Chennai alone. Alis are almost entirely dependent on sex work.

While most Alis are transsexuals,[6] they also include transvestites, some of who plan to undergo sex change operations. Alis have a high number of paid sexual contacts with 'heterosexual' men. They reside in fairly poor conditions (although there exists some variation in economic status between them) and cruise in particularly dark and unhygienic areas, such as on the banks of the polluted river Cooum, near railway tracks or in open grounds. They engage in a range of sexual practices including *sapti* (inter-femoral sex—between the thighs), anal and oral sex. All Alis are members of the Jamaath, or community, with some having recognised leadership, or *guru*, status. Cut off from their families and communities of origin, they lead a

communal existence in the neighbourhoods and suburbs of Chennai.
Alis are known to be geographically mobile within Tamil Nadu and
their yearly itineraries may include travel between Chennai,
Bangalore, Mumbai, Pune and, to a lesser extent, New Delhi.

Sexual Health Interventions for Men Who Have Sex with Men and Alis in Chennai

Through mapping the sexual geography of homosexual contacts as
well as the knowledge gained as a result of the situational assessment, a multifaceted intervention project for HIV prevention
among MSM was developed at the end of 1993. With the backing
of the National AIDS Control Organisation (NACO) and the State
AIDS Project Cell of Tamil Nadu, the Community Action Network
(CAN)[7] obtained technical and funding support through the GPA
for a 12-month project beginning in March 1994 (see Table 6.1),
which was subsequently extended for another period of 12 months.

Table 6.1
MSM Intervention, Chennai, Survey in August 1994

Variables	Intervention PSEs (n = 100) August 1994	Non-Intervention PSEs (n = 50) August 1994	Intervention PSEs (n = 225) 1995
Condom use in last sexual contact	52 (52%)	9 (18%)	65%
Project contact (by peer educators)	75 (75%)	2 (4%)	85%
Reporting only oral sex in last encounter	17 (17%)	NA	57%
Reporting only anal sex	78 (78%)	NA	38%

Outreach Encounters

MSM who have a good knowledge of the PSEs were recruited as outreach field staff. They were provided training in STD/AIDS prevention and in outreach, and their field work was well structured and regularly monitored. Outreach encounters initially focused on MSM who were regularly found at these locations but eventually expanded to their sexual partners or, in cases of prostitution, the clients, who were less easily identifiable. Emphasis was placed on reaching new persons but also on ensuring follow-up with previous contacts. Outreach encounters (see Table 6.2) usually included establishing rapport, informing about HIV/AIDS and providing condoms. Supportive IEC material was also provided and, when possible, outreach workers demonstrated correct condom use on models. Repeat contacts involved more detailed discussions about relative risk associated with sexual practices and, at times, the provision of referrals to health services.

Table 6.2
Number of Outreach Encounters, Condoms given
and Health Referrals Provided per Month

Indicators	August 1994	November 1994	January 1995	December 1995	December 1996
Numbers of outreach encounters	1,117	3,004	3,189	4,820	7,844
Number of new persons reached in outreach contacts	584	1,255	772	1,231	654
Number of condoms provided during outreach	6,449	8,551	8,477	13,342	21,345
Number of health referrals provided	49	40	78	114	122

The number of outreach encounters in August 1994 was 1,117 and went upto 7,844 by December 1996. There was strong focus on follow-up contacts and the outreach experience developed gradually, and an attempt is now being made to qualitatively improve and revise guidelines for outreach encounters—repeat contacts, for example, developed to deal with specific issues, such as STDs.

Condom Promotion and Distribution

Initially, outreach workers and other peer educators focused on promoting condom use in penetrative sex. Over the months these educators and other volunteers became part of an elaborate system of condom distribution for MSM. The uptake of condoms has been greatest among those involved in prostitution, as a direct association is now made between reduced incidence of STDs and the protective role of condoms. Near some PSEs, several points were selected for stocking condoms—in tea shops and stalls and with guards at parks.

While the project gives out free condoms, the distribution is need-based and on demand. In August 1994, 6,449 condoms were distributed, 8,477 by January 1995 and 21,345 by December 1996, showing the increased demand for condoms. Given the lack of financial resources among many MSM the project is likely to continue free distribution of condoms.

Health Services

As in most outreach-based projects referrals to health or other services is slow to evolve. In the context of MSM the issue of STDs was the most difficult to address. In addition, there was a need to inform MSM about where these services could be obtained and to reassure them that they would be well received by the health care workers. To this effect the project has not only focused its attention on the users of these services but has also addressed the way these services are provided in a number of health centres. The project established a formal relation with these services, discussed issues specific to the target population and accompanied persons to health services. Counsellors at the project office assured individual counselling when needed.

The use of peer members as health care facilitators ensured greater acceptance by treatment seekers and also helped service providers relate better with community members. The training on syndromic management of health care providers already being accessed by the community members also improved the quality of STD care provided by them.

The services at the general hospital where an Ali peer health worker received Ali community members ensured quick and good quality treatment, including treatment with respect, and the number of Alis seeking health care doubled in the first six months of 1996 and covered 97 per cent of the Ali community by December 1996. The attitude of the various health care providers also showed substantial change and for the first time they 'started seeing the human side of these people'.[8] This system had become functional for STD care and other health problems in early 1995.

Counselling

The project office has in many ways become a community drop-in centre for members of the target population and in this context, the role of the project counsellors is being evaluated. One of the functions has been to interface between health services, including HIV testing centres, and the population. The project has also supported activities for those who are HIV seropositive.

However, the long-term need for these services is difficult to evaluate at present. Among certain subpopulations, such as trans-sexual prostitutes, the knowledge that a number are HIV+ will probably be a determining factor in changes in norms around sexual practices.

The Gay Movement in India and HIV/AIDS Interventions

The gay movement in India is still at a nascent stage. While homosexuality has an ancient history—descriptions of same-sex relationships in the Kama Sutra, women loving women in the Mahabharata and the Ramayana, court customs of Babar, Hindu festivals and sects that celebrate homosexuality (Mukherjee 1990)—'gay' as a political identity is still emerging.

The emergence of the identity is still shrouded and, from a state of namelessness, it has appropriated and subverted languages which have been integral to the invention of the identity. The first South Asian newsletter on homosexuality was named Anamika, which in Sanskrit means 'nameless'.

However, gay bashing by the police and by heterosexuals has been reported. In 1994, the National Federation of Indian Women (NFIW)—a women's organisation affiliated to the Communist Party of India (CPI)—expressed outrage against the South Asian Gay Conferences in Mumbai, describing it as an invasion of India by decadent Western cultures.

The AIDS pandemic has made homophobia a more serious problem. AIDS was and, in many parts, still is considered to be a homosexual disease. MSM also undergo heterosexism—prejudice or discrimination against gay people. One of the ways to counter the inferior status of gays was to bring into the limelight eminent gay personalities who were open about their sexuality. At times this has also led to 'outing', or forcible hounding and exposing, of gay people who were unwilling to publicly admit their sexual orientation.

The public movement towards the rights of gays and lesbians in India was put forth in an organised manner at the end of 1991 through the charter of demands which contains 19 elements and was published in the last chapter of the report 'Less Than Gay' and includes demands to repeal discriminatory legislation, including Section 377 of the IPC. In 1992, a demonstration was held in New Delhi to protest against police atrocities against homosexuals. This was followed by moving a petition in the petitions committee of the parliament, which is still pending.

While the public movement towards sexual liberation is ongoing, there is a move towards organising the community and developing support systems for those who have an alternate sexuality. There are at least 10 active gay groups in the country, with many of them having widely subscribed publications. Many of them organise regular meetings for their members.

Apart from this, parties and social gathering form another part of the gay culture. Sneha Sangama in 1993 and 1996 at Bangalore, Goan Utsav 1993, Masti 1994 at Jaipur, Big Bash in 1994 and new year parties in Mumbai and Kolkata are examples of large get-togethers. Gays and lesbians have strong networks at local levels as well as at the national level.

The network of gay groups in India has perhaps not taken on issues around HIV/AIDS as much as their counterparts in the West. This is due to various limitations, including not wanting to reinforce the stigma of HIV. But a lot of change has come about over the last few years. From a stage when a worker promoting condoms during one of the gay get-togethers in 1993 was physically attacked and thrown out, active support for HIV prevention is today a key focus for most. Most of the gay publications, including Bombay Dost, Fun Club, Aarambh, Sakhi, Khush Club, Good As You, Men India Movement, Sisters, Udaan, Saathi, Gay Information Centre, carry or provide information on HIV/AIDS. Condom promotion through networks and advertisement is also undertaken.

The Humsafar Trust, Mumbai, runs a drop-in centre which 'creates a dynamic interface between the target groups and the public health services' (Kavi 1996). The centre has been functioning since October 1995 and has a weekly attendance of approximately 50 men. Between October 1995 and January 1996, the centre had registered 340 individual interventions, distributed 9,000 condoms, conducted 17 workshops and trained 10 volunteers for street outreach.

The Naz project in Kolkata mapped 17 public sex sites and has started providing on-site one-to-one information dissemination and counselling, including subsidised STD/HIV testing and treatment for STDs. The Naz Foundation (India) Trust in Delhi also targets male commercial sex workers and their male clients. The programme includes STD treatment and basic health care, counselling and addresses issues related to sexual identity.

Given the high prevalence of MSM activity, the services available to them and interventions addressing them are grossly inadequate. National AIDS programmes rarely incorporate the needs of men who have sex with men. In a survey conducted by PANOS amongst ASOs, NGOs and gay organisations and individuals 65 per cent of the respondents felt that the issue of MSM and HIV was not consistently acknowledged (PANOS 1997). Funding for work with MSM has also not been forthcoming. Although it is clear to many that male-to-male sex plays an important role in India's epidemic of AIDS, the country's AIDS prevention budget for 1992–96, laid down in the strategic plan for the prevention and control of AIDS in India exemplifies the problems of funding prevention activities targeted at men who have sex with men. The five-year budget allows for a total expenditure of just US$350,000 for HIV prevention work among this group compared to US$25 million for work among female prostitutes (Ministry of Health and Family Welfare 1992). This also has a negative impact as most of the IEC messages focus on the heterosexual route and often imply that one can get infected if 'you have sex with a prostitute'.[9] This reinforces the belief among many of the MSM community members that AIDS, like other STDs, is a 'pombale noi', or women's disease, that you get from women and that male-to-male sex indeed protects them from HIV/AIDS.

Discussion

While it is clear that there is a substantial population of MSM in India, interventions addressing the needs of this community are grossly inadequate. While the interventions that have been developed in the country clearly show that it is possible to have effective interventions with the MSM community, a number of important lessons that emerge need to be kept in mind while designing interventions with MSM.

What are the strategies that work with the MSM community? The answer to this is not simple, though some generalisations can be made. While the work of CAN and that of others· addressing the MSM community has focused on outreach and service provision at PSEs, the work with Alis in Chennai has taken on a community development approach, with HIV as a focus area. It has looked at empowerment of the community members through literacy, skill building, additional income generation to minimise dependence on selling sex, advocacy with others, including the police, and working with the media to raise awareness about the community and thereby created an enabling environment. Thus the needs of the communities being addressed would vary from place to place and from situation to situation. Overall, the consensus seems to emerge that interventions should use both enabling and persuasive strategies to be effective. Behaviour change communication focusing on one-to-one education, outreach at PSEs, providing access to good quality condoms and skills in condom usage, facilitation of improved sexual health service to guarantee respectful and non-stigmatizing treatment, counselling and advocacy to minimise homophobia are the broad strategies that have been found to be effective.

The need to provide choices to the members of the community is also an important factor in the success of any intervention. A question that has often been asked concerns the need for promoting oral and other less risky practices, such as, mutual masturbation and what is known in the MSM and Ali circuits as *sapti* sex. On one side are the moralists who question whether attempts to promote such practices encourages 'amoral' behaviour, while, on the other, there is a debate about how safe oral sex is. The CAN project's response has been that oral sex is certainly less risky than anal sex. As to the moral question, people have a right to their own choices and the project's responsibility is to ensure that the risk involved is minimised.

The divide between the gay community as it is understood in the West and the reality of MSM in the Indian context should be kept in mind while designing interventions. Class divides are very high in the MSM circuit and often there is outright hatred of MSM from the lower classes (who form the bulk of the MSM community) by MSM from the middle and upper middle classes who identify themselves as truly gay. One of the primary reasons for this is that MSM from the lower classes may resort to commercial MSM activity which is looked down upon by those from the higher classes. In the first two months of the project CAN organised dance parties to attract MSM community members and to reach out to them with messages about the project and about sexual health. One of the expensive lessons learnt during this period was that the parties attracted only MSM members from the upper middle class. The other MSM members refused to come and one of them put very succinctly the reason why he did not attend. 'The Coke and beer culture alienates the bulk of the MSM as many are ordinary lower class people who do not go to these hotels and are very uncomfortable in these posh settings.' It is also clear that men who have sex with men are likely to vary considerably in terms of their attitudes towards their own sexuality, sexual practices and their desire for visibility or anonymity (Gordon 1996). It is not uncommon to see many of the lower and middle class men from the MSM groups getting married. It is often a social obligation that they cannot escape.[10]

Another issue that has to considered is the ownership of the interventions. While there has been a lot of debate about the need to have communities take on the ownership of the project, it is still unclear as to how effective the strategy will be, given the social stigma and marginalisation. One of the key debates that has been ongoing and has often been led by the donors has been the need to have communities take charge of the projects. This is often not supported by enough attempts to enable and equip the communities to undertake the management of the projects, leading to the collapse of the projects once the agencies withdraw. This has been seen in a number of cases and the example of CAN is another that shows the collapse of a good intervention because of the agenda to withdraw and let the communities take charge.[11] While it is crucial to have community members play a lead role in the development and management of interventions, there is first a need to develop the capacities of the community members to handle the responsibility.

The key factor that needs to be understood by policy makers and implementers is that there is a sizeable population of MSM who have relatively low levels of awareness, lower access to health care services and minimal level of risk perception. Many of them are bisexual and thus could be passing on their infections to their wives/heterosexual partners.

What is urgently needed is a realistic look at the issues surrounding male-to-male sex and its implications for HIV transmission. While there are clear indications that male-to-male sex in India is as much or as low as in any other culture, research can provide greater insights into its spread and construction in the Indian context. The decision as to whether there should be interventions for MSM should, however, be based on the reality that emerges, rather than on assumptions.

Notes

1. This is often because the available epidemiological categories (heterosexual, homosexual and bisexual) are not culturally relevant and, therefore, meaningful. Due to social stigma and ramifications men may be very reluctant to admit to anal intercourse with other men. See also McKenna 1996.
2. Bombay Dost, Stree Sangam and Humsafar Trust in Mumbai, Counsel Club, Sappho and Pravartak in Kolkata, Good as You and Sangama in Bangalore, Saathi in Hyderabad, OLAVA in Pune and Arambh in New Delhi, to name a few.
3. A study by the Naz Foundation (India) Trust in 1996 revealed that 90 per cent of the clients of male sex workers were married. Few, if any, of the wives of

these men knew of their husbands' sex with other men. Thirty-five per cent of the respondents of the Naz study reported having anal sex with their wives.

4. For example, in Morocco (Boushaba 1994) or Braxil (Guimaraes et al. 1994), a belief shared by many men who have had sex with other men and one that is implicitly accepted by the societies in which they live is that the insertive partner in anal intercourse is not in any way deviating from the norms of expected and acceptable masculine behaviour. The active partner carries no stigma, no shame, no consciousness of social or sexual deviation, allowing him to see himself and be seen as completely heterosexual. All the burden of a deviant—invariably shameful, probably criminal—sexual behaviour and identity is carried by the receptive or passive partner in anal intercourse.

5. Observation and key informant interviews resulted in the identification of more than 70 PSEs of different sizes across the city. An inventory carried out at all these PSEs provided the estimate of the number of MSM who regularly visit these sites. The estimate is also based on the number of new outreach contacts made by the project workers during the intervention.

6. Most Alis in Chennai have undergone castration, or attained *nirvana*. The process of castration could be through a traditional *dayamma*, who may use a crude method for removing the genitals or, more recently, through qualified medical practitioners, mostly in Pune and Dindugal, near Chennai. It is for this reason that they are often referred to as eunuchs by those familiar with Western discourse. The word eunuch is not an adequate term as it is used to mark men who are emasculated. It says nothing about the gender identity of this person. Mogul rulers made use of eunuchs to guard their harems. Often these men were emasculated but continued to have a masculine identity. The word Ali or Hijra always refers to gender status.

7. CAN is a community-based NGO which implements targeted interventions for HIV/AIDS with female sex workers and their clients, with MSM and with the Ali community in Chennai. The WHO–GPA study on MSM circuits in 1993 was carried out by researchers affiliated to CAN.

8. 'Earlier when we used to come here, we had to wait till all others were finished with their treatment. Then the doctors would ask us to strip and take photographs, call 20 students and we would be exhibits. It was better to suffer the pain than to go through this humiliation. We would not come till it [pain] became unbearable. Now things are better. Noori [peer health worker] is there to take care and the people are more understanding'—field notes, CAN.

9. One of the key factors that helped the project reach out to MSM with the message on AIDS in their community was the role played by Sekhar, a member of the MSM community who was living with HIV. In the initial phase of the project, MSM community members believed that HIV was not an issue that they needed to be worried about as they 'never had sex with prostitutes'. This was because most of the AIDS prevention messages that were being given out by the government claimed that one could get infected with the virus through sex with prostitutes. It was only after Sekhar came out in the open with his HIV status that the community started responding to AIDS messages, especially as they knew Sekhar well and knew that he had never had sex with a woman in his life, and was still infected. It was also during this period that Vidya (name changed), an Ali, died due to AIDS. This had an impact on the MSM and Ali communities and for the first time they realised that there was HIV amidst them.

10. During the last three years of my work with the MSM community, of the 12 field workers in the office four have got married. 'None of us can escape marriage. It is essential.' There was one of my field workers whose parents found out that he had sex with men and thought that marriage was the answer. He ran away from home and went to Mumbai and joined a group of Hijras and is now saving money to undergo castration. The first reaction of parents who find that their son is part of the MSM community is to force him into marriage. This also shows the continuum of the MSM-to-women transmission.

11. An attempt is underway to hand over the projects to the community members to take overall charge. This has not been successful as the members expressed lack of experience and unwillingness to take on the administrative burden 'as it is too early'.

References/Further Reading

Arvind, K., 1991. *Invisible Minority*. Bombay: Dynamic.

Devi, S., 1977. *The World of homosexuals*. New Delhi: Vikas Publishing House.

Gordon, Peter, 1996. *Review of 'Best Practice' for Targeted Interventions*.

ICMR, 1992. 'HIV Infections: Current Dimensions and Future Implications'. *ICMR Bulletin*, 22: 11–12.

John, T.J. et al., 1993. 'The Epidemiology of AIDS in the Vellore Region, Southern India'. *AIDS*, 7: 412–24.

Ministry of Health and Family Welfare, 1992. *Strategic Plan for the Prevention and Control of AIDS in India, 1992–1996*. New Delhi: Ministry of Health and Family Welfare.

McKenna, Neil, 1996. *On the Margins: Men Who Have Sex with Men and HIV in the Developing World*. PANOS.

Mukherjee, Subodh, 1990. *Trikone*, 5: 1.

Nandi, Jayashree, Hemant Kamat, Varsha Bhavalkar and Kalyan Banerjee, 1994. 'Detection of Human Immunodeficiency Virus Antibody among Homosexual Men from Bombay'. *Sexually Transmitted Diseases*, 235–36.

National AIDS Control Programme, Tamil Nadu State AIDS Project Cell and WHO/Global Program on AIDS, 1993. 'Men Who Have Sex with Men: Assessment of situation in Madras'. Confidential report.

Orton, L., 1995. 'Special Survey: Tamil Nadu and Madras'. *AIDS Analysis*, 1(1): 3–9.

PANOS, 1997. *On the Margins*, Chapter 9, page 86.

Row Kavi, Ashoke, 1991. 'AIDS Action International Newsletter on AIDS Prevention and Control'. 15: 4.

Row Kavi, Asoke, 1996. 'STD/HIV Prevention Program in Bombay's Emerging Gay Community and AIDS Outreach in the Men Who Have Sex with Men Sector'. Paper presented at the XI International AIDS Conference, Vancouver.

Tan, Michael L., 1994. 'Recent HIV/AIDS Trends among Men Who Have Sex with Men'. Yokohoma Conference Paper PL-13.

7

Targeted Intervention in Injecting Drug Users: Some Experiences

Anindya Chatterjee, M. Suresh Kumar
and *Abu S. Abdul-Quader*

Introduction

This chapter focuses on HIV prevention interventions targeting injecting drug users (IDUs). It begins with brief descriptions of interventions that have been implemented in different parts of the world. Then we describe a number of interventions that have been implemented in India. Instead of attempting to summarise all the interventions, we give brief descriptions of selected interventions that have been implemented in four different regions of the country. Next we discuss the problems and barriers encountered in implementing these interventions. In the concluding section, we focus on the lessons learned and examine the feasibility of such interventions in India.

There are a number of reasons for preventing transmission of HIV/AIDS among drug injectors. HIV infections among IDUs has become a worldwide public health problem. By 1996, drug injection has been reported in 120 countries and HIV infection among drug injectors in over 80 of these countries (Des Jarlais et al. 1996). The latter is a substantial increase over the 59 countries with HIV infection among IDUs in 1989 (Des Jarlais and Friedman 1989).

Several factors have been associated with the extremely rapid transmission of HIV among IDUs—(1) lack of awareness of HIV/AIDS as a local threat; (2) restrictions on the availability and use of new injecting equipment; and (3) mechanisms for rapid, efficient mixing within local IDU populations. Without an awareness of AIDS as a local threat, injecting drug users are likely to use each other's equipment very frequently.

Legal restrictions can reduce the availability of sterile injecting equipment and thus lead to increased multiperson use (sharing) of drug injecting equipment. In some jurisdictions, medical prescriptions are required for the purchase of needles and syringes. Possession of needles and syringes can also be criminalised as 'drug paraphernalia', putting users at risk of arrest if needles and syringes are found in their possession. Drug users have also been prosecuted in some jurisdictions for possession, based on the minute quantities of drugs that remain in a needle and syringe after it has been used to inject. In addition to the possible legal restrictions on the availability of sterile injecting equipment, the actual practices of pharmacists and the police can create important limits. Even if laws permit the sale of needles and syringes without prescriptions, pharmacists may choose not to sell without prescriptions, or not to sell to anyone who 'looks like a drug user'. Similarly, the police may harass drug users found carrying injecting equipment even if there are no laws criminalising the possession of narcotics paraphernalia.

Simple sharing of needles and syringes among sexual partners or small groups of friends is not sufficient to cause an epidemic of rapid HIV transmission among IDUs. For rapid transmission to occur, there needs to be some mechanism by which large numbers of IDUs can share equipment with each other within relatively short time periods. Shooting galleries (places where IDUs can rent injecting equipment, which is then returned to gallery owners for rental to other IDUs) and dealers' works (injecting equipment kept by a drug seller, which can be lent for successive drug purchases) are examples of situations that provide the possibility of rapid transmission of HIV among IDUs. In many cities, IDUs will gather at specific locations, form loose groups to purchase drugs (better prices can usually be obtained if users purchase in large volumes) and then inject together, sharing the injecting equipment. Membership in these drug purchasing groups will then change very rapidly. Several studies have indicated that the infectiousness of HIV is many times greater in the two-to-three month period after initial infection compared to the long latency period between initial infection and the development of severe immunosuppression. Thus, the concentration of new infections in these settings may synergistically interact with continued mixing and lead to highly infectious IDUs transmitting HIV to large numbers of other drug injectors.

Several other factors may also facilitate the sharing of injecting equipment. For example, in some countries, injecting is the only way for many people to begin using drugs and, sometimes, drugs are only available in injectable forms. Further, high rates of polysubstance use may lead to intoxication with alcohol or other drugs prior to injecting, which increases the liklihood of sharing 'dirty works'.

Besides through sharing of injecting equipment, HIV is also transmitted and acquired through unprotected sexual intercourse. Among many people who use recreational drugs, periods of drug use are likely to be interspersed with phases comprising conventional behaviour, including sexual activity. The risk of transmission of HIV through sex with an IDU is closely related to the frequency of equipment sharing, the frequency of risk-associated sexual activity and also to the extent of the epidemic in a given area.

HIV Interventions Targeting Injecting Drug Users

In response to the problem of HIV transmission among IDUs, a variety of prevention interventions have been implemented in different parts of the world. These interventions have been found to be effective in reducing as well as preventing transmission of HIV. A substantial body of empirical and theoretical evidence demonstrates that a reduction in the sharing of injection drug use equipment significantly reduces HIV transmission rates among IDUs. The following discussion presents brief summaries of some of the interventions used with IDUs.

Education of IDUs

One of the interventions that can facilitate risk reduction is education of IDUs to raise their awareness about the risk of contracting HIV through injection drug use. Studies conducted in the United States have shown the positive impact of educational programmes targeting IDUs (Ostrow 1989). In contrast, the impact of a lack of basic factual information about HIV/AIDS can be seen in the very rapid spread of HIV in many areas of Southeast Asia where little AIDS education occurred prior to the initial, rapid spread of HIV among IDUs.

Increasing Availability of Clean Injecting Equipment

Making available clean needles and syringes is the most controversial measure so far taken in attempting to prevent HIV among IDUs. Clean needles and syringes can be made available to IDUs through needle and syringes exchange programmes, pharmacy-based programmes or pharmacy sale of needles and syringes. Secondary outlets, such as health centres, drug dealers, vending machines and outreach distribution, could be used as well. Because of legal restrictions in many countries, it has been very difficult to implement needle exchange programmes.

Evaluation of needle exchange programmes around the world shows that they have played a significant role in lowering the rates of needle sharing among IDUs (Institute for Health Policy Studies 1993, Hartgers et al. 1989, Stimson 1989, Des Jarlais and Maynard 1992) and have served as referral sources for other health related services (Dolan et al. 1993). Needle exchange programmes have also been found *not* to lead to an increase in drug use *nor* an increase in HIV drug-risk behaviours. Furthermore, HIV infection rates in many cities have remained stable after implementation of needle exchange programmes.

Decontamination of Used Needles and Syringes

There are two effective approaches to de-activate HIV in injecting equipment—heat and chemicals. Continuous boiling in water for 20 minutes is sufficient to render HIV inactive. However, this may not be a practical option for many IDUs. An alternative is decontamination using a bleach solution. Bleach is strong and easily available, and it harm's neither the injecting equipment nor the injector. Bleach distribution programmes were first initiated in

San Francisco and later in other cities in the USA. The use of bleach was generally accepted by IDUs and, in the absence of syringe exchange programmes, bleach was used by a large proportion of IDUs where it was distributed.

Although bleach is easily available and accepted by the IDUs, studies in the USA have failed to show any relationship between self-reported use of bleach to disinfect injecting equipment and protection from infection with HIV (Vlahov et al. 1994, Titus et al. 1994). Several other factors may also determine the efficacy of bleach in protecting IDUs from HIV infection. First, the drug users may not know how to 'properly' use bleach to disinfect injecting equipment. Second, even if the drug users know how to properly use bleach, they may not be doing so under 'field conditions' (Gleghorn et al. 1994). The chemical strength of bleach varies from country to country, and it is the free-chlorine concentration in such solutions that governs effectiveness against HIV.

Pharmacological Treatment of Drug Addiction

There are now numerous studies that have demonstrated that participation in pharmacological maintenance treatment, such as methadone maintenance, reduces HIV transmission and acquisition. It has been shown, for example, that risk-associated behaviour, incidence of new HIV infection and overall HIV seroprevalence are significantly lower in IDUs undergoing methadone maintenance treatment than among those not being treated (Caplehorn and Ross 1995).

Outreach as a Method of Intervention

Since the beginning of the AIDS epidemic, outreach has been initiated in the United States and later in other countries to educate IDUs about HIV infection and to encourage them to engage in HIV risk-reduction behaviours. The outreach programmes have provided HIV/AIDS prevention information-education materials to IDUs and established links with available services such as drug treatment, HIV counselling and testing, medical care and social services. The programmes often provide some means for engaging in risk-reduction behaviours, such as clean syringes, bleach for decontaminating used syringes and condoms for safer sexual behaviour. Most of these programmes have hired ex-drug users as peer outreach workers. These outreach interventions have been found to be effective both in reaching IDUs who had never been in any drug treatment programmes and in reducing HIV risk behaviours (Abdul-Quader et al. 1992, MMWR 1993, Neaigus et al. 1990, Weibel et al. 1993).

HIV Testing

The role of HIV testing in prevention is not conclusive. Studies conducted in the United States and other countries have shown that while testing for HIV may have contributed to the prevention of HIV/AIDS among the general population, the effect among IDUs was not conclusive. In order to use testing for prevention purposes, appropriate counselling must accompany testing. In addition, issues such as anonymity and confidentiality are also important (Cartter et al. 1990, Higgins et al. 1991).

Organisation of IDUs

Establishing organisations of IDUs can have a considerable positive impact in communities where individual IDUs are reluctant to identify themselves because of the legal or stigmatising environment. In some countries, drug users' organisations have been found to be very helpful in the fight against HIV/AIDS.

The drug users' organisation can organise provision of services, such as needle and syringe exchange, have significant community advocacy role, provide advice to health departments and be a good source of information for IDUs. It involves users and ex-users, therefore, maintains close relations with the whole IDU community. This is also a good way to mobilise support and enthusiasm. They also act as entry points to other active users.

Social Network Interventions:
Case Studies from Different Cities in India

There is a wide difference in HIV seroprevalence among IDUs in India. In the north-eastern state of Manipur, where HIV among IDUs was first reported in 1989, seroprevalence among IDUs is the highest—about 80 per cent. Chennai in the south has reported about 30 per cent seroprevalence among IDUs. The seroprevalence in Kolkata is about 1 per cent. HIV has also been reported among alcohol users in Bangalore. Responses to the epidemic have been varied depending on the extent of the problem as well as the avail-ability of resources and the political will of the larger community. Since late 1980s and early 1990s, a variety of intervention pro-grammes targeting the IDUs have been initiated in different parts of the country. In the following pages we describe a number of interventions that have been implemented in different parts of the country. We do *not* make an attempt to provide a comprehensive overview of the interventions that have been implemented. Rather, examples of interventions implemented in certain parts of the country are described.

Interventions Targeting IDUs in Manipur

Background

Manipur has been the focus of national and international atten-tion since HIV was first reported among IDUs there in 1989. Over 80 per cent of the IDUs in Manipur are estimated to be HIV+ (ICMR 1992–95). One per cent of the antenatal mothers screened in the maternity clinics have been found to be HIV+ (ibid.). Mother-to-child transmission in the state has also been documented (Panda et al. 1994).

Manipur is estimated to have about 20,000 injectors. Since 1989, a variety of intervention activities have been initiated in the state by different non-governmental organisations (NGOs) and the Indian Council of Medical Research. Initially, the interven-tions were limited to drug treatment which was based on spiritual healing and other non-pharmacological interventions. Most of the treatment centres have been set up by NGOs established by ex-users. They also provided limited drug and HIV risk-reduction counselling. A major focus of the intervention has been psycho-social counselling rather than behavioural risk reduction. At the same time these organisations also initiated outreach to IDUs—especially HIV+ IDUs. ICMR, as part of its research efforts, also conducted outreach to IDUs at their homes and in the local prisons where they were kept by the authorities.

While most of these activities have been initiated by a variety of government and non-governmental organisations, very few have attempted a systematic evaluation of activities. In 1994, the WHO funded and supported an outreach intervention programme targeting the IDUs in Churachandpur and this was the first such intervention in the state of Manipur. This programme was implemented in the town of Churachandpur (population 40,000) with 600 to 800 IDUs. It is 66 km from Imphal, the state capital and the communication facilities are poor. There are nine major ethnic groups in Churachandpur and as many dialects. Christianity is the dominant religion. In spite of this diverse ethnicity, the different dialects are widely understood and the groups share a common way of life. Economic underdevelopment has meant that the community has retained its agrarian way of life, where women work along with men. Most live in extended families; the church and community leaders have a major influence in the community. Unemployment is very high. The town has a heavy military presence due to the underground political groups in the area which are engaged in armed struggle for self-rule.

In Churachandpur, herion injection began in the early 1980s. Most of the heroin came from Myanmar. The town's six drug treatment centres, which are run by voluntary workers, ex-users and doctors, use spiritual and 12-step treatment programmes. No maintenance treatment is available, abstinence from drugs being the only behavioural goal. Some IDUs have shifted to injecting dextropropoxyphene, which is cheap and easily available, and the number of new dextropropoxyphene injectors has been growing.

Implementation of the Outreach Project

The major objective of the project was to assess the feasibility of implementing an intervention targeting IDUs and measure its efficacy in reducing risks of HIV infection. The intervention includes a number of components. These are (a) street-based outreach to drug users and their sex partners; (b) distribution of information-education and risk-reduction materials; (c) outreach to family members and friends of IDUs and members of the community; (d) advocacy with the administration, law enforcement authorities, church organisations and other community-based organisations; (e) drug treatment referrals; (f) medical treatment for minor ailments and referrals to hospitals; and (g) outreach at dealers' places.

The project recruited and trained a number of ex-users as outreach workers and a number of current users as volunteers to provide HIV/AIDS risk-reduction information and education, distribute risk-reduction materials such as condoms and bleach. One of the innovative strategies were to recruit current drug users and train them to disseminate HIV/AIDS prevention information to IDUs and shooting gallery owners. They also distributed risk-reduction materials to shooting gallery owners.

Periodic cross-sectional surveys of IDUs were conducted to measure changes in risk behaviours and initiation of risk reduction by IDUs. Data indicated that the project has not only fulfilled the objectives in terms of implementation of outreach in a developing country setting and in reaching a majority of the IDUs in Churachandpur, it has also been successful in initiating risk reduction among IDUs (Hangzo et al. 1997). There has been a significant increase in the proportion of IDUs mentioned to have received HIV/AIDS risk-reduction materials (39 to 76 per cent), talked to someone about HIV/AIDS (42 to 61 per cent), and have someone talk to them (51 to 84 per cent). Seventy-eight per cent of the IDUs mentioned to have initiated HIV/AIDS risk reduction, compared to 59 per cent during the first survey. Ever use of bleach increased from 31 per cent to 72 per cent after one year (Chatterjee et al. 1996).

While the project made significant contributions in terms of implementation of an outreach intervention in a high drug-use developing country setting and helped in initiation of risk reduction, a number of problems which require attention by the authorities remain. For example, even though there has been an increase in the use of bleach, it has not been consistent. This has been because bleach was not always available, it has been difficult for IDUs to carry bleach, and because of the searches carried out by the police. Similarly, while there has been a change in the proportion of IDUs mentioned to have initiated HIV/AIDS risk reduction, sharing of syringe and needle has not yet changed. This has been due to the fact that clean syringes and needles were not available and they were difficult to carry because of police searches of IDUs.

In addition to this project in Churachandpur, a number of NGOs have also initiated HIV prevention interventions targeting IDUs in Manipur. A needle exchange programme was set up by SHALOM, a local NGO in Churachandpur. Three other NGOs supported and funded by Swedish Sida have started needle exchange programmes in Imphal. As the programmes have not yet been evaluated, their impact could not be measured. A number of the local NGOs in Imphal have been involved in providing HIV/AIDS risk-reduction information and education to IDUs. They also provide domiciliary care to HIV-infected IDUs.

While voluntary HIV testing has been offered to IDUs, there was mandatory testing of drug users in jail and the test results were declared with photographs in the local newspapers. Voluntary testing for HIV became very unpopular and only a very small percentage (10–15 per cent) of those tested returned to find out the test results.

Interventions Targeting IDUs in Chennai

Background

Since 1983, Chennai has been experiencing a rise in heroin use and, since 1991, injection use of buprenrophine has also been steadily increasing. Easy availability of injectable preparations such as buprenrophine has contributed to this increase. It has been estimated that there are about 15,000 injecting drug users in Chennai. IDUs have been seen in a number of different locations in the city. A number of estimates of HIV prevalence in Chennai have been put forth with samples from drug treatment centres and voluntary testing facilities. Prevalence of HIV has been found to be between 15 and 20 per cent. In addition to HIV, prevalence of HBV is also high among the IDUs in Chennai. It is estimated to be 37 per cent among buprenrophine injectors and 32 per cent among heroin injectors (Kumar et al. 1995). Findings from a 1995 study show that many of the drug users were unaware of the existing HIV testing facility in the city and most of them were reluctant to get tested for HIV (ibid).

Assessment conducted among street-recruited IDUs shows that sharing of injecting equipment was common. More than two-thirds of the IDUs interviewed claimed to have shared equipment in the one month prior to the interview (Kumar and Daniels 1994). Sometimes, needles were not shared but syringes were. In addition to sharing syringes and needles, sharing of the spoon and the drug solution, and of the cotton swab were very common. On an average, the heroin users injected two to four times a day as opposed to the buprenrophine users, who injected less frequently because of the longer effect on the drug.

There are a number of differences between heroin and buprenrophine users. Most heroin users were in touch with other users. Their networks were larger in size. Even though the ties and bondage changed over time, at any point in time, the heroin users had at least one or more drug users with whom they had a reciprocal relationship. The heroin users usually took the drug in the street and the places where drugs were sold also facilitated sharing. The setting encouraged sharing. In contrast, the buprenrophine networks were smaller and most had only one or two drug using persons in their network. Most of them lived with their families and the family members were supportive of the drug users (Kumar et al. 1995).

Casual and commercial sex were frequent among drug users in Chennai. Condom use was very low. Sexually transmitted infections were high and buprenrophine users reported more unprotected sexual encounters than heroin injectors (Kumar et al. 1995, Mudaliar and Kumar 1996).

HIV Interventions Targeting Drug Users in Chennai

In 1991, the first outreach services were set up by SAHAI Trust, an organisation involved in the treatment of drug users. The outreach team consisted of ex-users and professional social workers. The team conducted street outreach and provided HIV/AIDS education and information, and information on decontamination of syringes and needles. The workers also distributed bleach and condoms. Initially, the outreach intervention was individually targeted and later, changing peer and social norms were emphasised. Increasingly, the drug users' networks were targeted.

Even though syringes were available in pharmacies without prescriptions and at a low cost, most IDUs continued to reuse, lend and borrow syringes. SAHAI Trust set up a syringe exchange programme to examine the feasibility of distributing syringes to

IDUs as well as the reaction of the community vis-à-vis syringe exchange. However, the programme is yet to be evaluated to assess feasibility and measure impact on risk behaviour.

A study conducted on risk behaviour indicates that drug users are making an effort to decrease their risks of getting infected with HIV. Use of buprenrophine itself can reduce risk, as buprenrophine users are likely to inject less, share less, have smaller sharing networks and share less injecting paraphernalia. Ethnographic information indicates that sharing of injecting equipment has decreased considerably and injectors do not share equipment when blood is visible in syringes. Many injectors have their own equipment. They are less likely to share with someone unknown to them. While drug risk behaviours decreased considerably, condom use remained very low.

Interventions Targeting IDUs in Delhi

Delhi has a relatively large drug using population. The majority of the users either smoke heroin or inject buprenrophine. However, very few interventions have been initiated in Delhi targeting the IDUs in the city. SHARAN—a Delhi based non-governmental organisation working for the urban poor—has initiated a substitution programme where drug users are offered oral buprenrophine as a substitute for heroin and injecting.

The project has been in operation since the beginning of 1995 and has so far attracted a large number of drug users. It initially started as an outreach service to the urban poor in Delhi and later on developed into a full-fledged intervention that included health education, information-education about HIV/AIDS, HIV/AIDS counselling and testing and also drug awareness among those who lived in the slums. Providing oral buprenrophine to injectors was not initially the project goal.

While providing outreach services, especially information on drug addiction, it became apparent that total abstinence may not be a practical goal for some of the drug users and that, for them, the focus should be more on risk reduction rather than on complete elimination of risks. Those who injected buprenrophine or heroin also took the risks of getting infected with HIV and other blood-borne pathogens. Providing oral buprenrophine to them may, it seemed, minimise their risks of getting infected with

HIV and other viruses, along with providing them with HIV risk-reduction information and education.

The project has not yet been formally evaluated. However, preliminary assessment and an evaluation conducted by Panda and Chatterjee (1997) show that the project has been successful in reaching a large number of drug users in Delhi and providing them with a variety of services, including substitution therapy. The project has so far reached 800 drug users within one and a half years, and about a third (about 300) of them have been maintained on oral buprenrophine.

The project has had modest success in reaching a large number of drug users in Delhi and providing them information on HIV/AIDS, health issues and also making them aware of drug use and abuse. The most significant outcome of the project is the establishment of oral buprenrophine not only as a substitute but also as a measure for preventing HIV/AIDS among IDUs.

Interventions Targeting IDUs in Kolkata

HIV among IDUs was initially thought to be a problem restricted to the north-eastern parts of the country. While a policy was introduced for testing the commercial sex workers (CSWs) in Kolkata and an intervention targeting the CSWs was subsequently implemented, no major attempt was made until very recently to address issues related to injection drug use and its risks for HIV transmission.

Similar to other metropolitan cities like Delhi and Chennai, Kolkata also had a large number of people smoking heroin. Coinciding with a decrease in street supply and rising cost of heroin, a significant proportion of heroin smokes in Kolkata switched over to injecting buprenorphine (Panda et al. 1997). The estimated prevalence of narcotic drug use in a few inner wards of the city was 0.3–0.5 per cent among the general population. The prevalence figure for the male population was 0.5–0.7 per cent, since this was largely a male problem (ICMR Report 1996). In this community-based study, it was also revealed that 60 per cent of the narcotic drug users were injectors. Needles were reportedly shared by 80 per cent (when last time injected) of the street-recruited IDUs. Sharing other paraphernalia such as the drug solution, rinse water and water container was universal. One of the methods of sharing the drug solution was known as 'syndicate' in the streets. When money was not enough to buy a whole 2 ml ampule of buprenorphine, drug injectors would put their money together. Often the same syringe or a multi-dose vial of chlorpheniramine was used to share the drug solution among the 'syndicate' of drug injectors. Buprenorphine was also cocktailed with other injectable such as chlorpheniramine, promethazine or diazepam to potentiate its effects. Injecting in deep veins, commonly the femoral veins, was used when the superficial veins get destroyed. More than half of the injectors had a history of abscess at the injecting site due to their habits of not cleaning the injecting site, keeping the drug solution in the syringe for a long time and not cleaning the syringe and the needle adequately. The common practice was to clean it with available water. About 15 per cent of the narcotic drug users also had suffered from tuberculosis.

HIV prevalence was found to be 1 per cent and the prevalence for hepatitis B was 18.5 per cent among the sample of IDUs. Sex in brothels with sex workers was quite common. Consistent condom use was non-existent (Panda et al. 1998).

The network of IDUs varied in size. In some areas of the city, it consisted of 5–10 individuals. In others there were many IDUs with homeless people. There was also a high degree of criminalisation, with drug users involved in petty crimes such as stealing, pickpocketing or sometimes working as agents of drug peddlers.

The city has a few drug treatment programmes mostly run by NGOs, which aim at abstinence as the only treatment goal. The number of in-patient treatment slots including rehabilitation programmes and meagre facilities at government mental hospitals are not more than 150. There were no substitution programmes except for the sublingual buprenorphine substitution from December 1999 to March 2001. It was found quite difficult to enrol a drug user from the streets into a drug treatment programme. All drug treatment programmes require some money either as treatment costs or cost of food which makes accessing drug treatment difficult.

Needle Exchange in Kolkata

Until recently there were no functional needle-exchange or HIV risk-reduction programmes. One of the NGOs runs a small needle-exchange programme not as an HIV-prevention activity but mainly to attract drug users in treatment.

The programme described here originated out of a research project of the Indian Council of Medical Research. It is primarily run by current drug using outreach staff who reaches out to IDUs everyday. There was also support from the general community for the project which developed over time. In addition to the street-based outreach, drop-in centres also provide support to outreach activities. The programme reached to about 300 IDUs of the city. The major components of the programme were:

1. Street-based outreach by drug user outreach workers
2. Peer education
3. Needle exchange
4. Distribution of other risk-reduction materials such as antiseptic cotton wipes, bleach, condoms, information materials
5. Dressing for abscess and limited facilities for primary health care
6. Drug treatment referral
7. STD/RTI treatment referral

The monitoring data from the project shows that a regular attender of the programme gets about three syringes and needles per week plus extra needles and other risk-reduction materials. At least half of those in the programme had stopped sharing needles (compared to 80 per cent at baseline rate one year back). This was also one of the economical programmes run primarily by drug users. The costs of the programme was around US$700 a month which clearly showed that needle-exchange programmes were cheap and could easily be implemented in Indian settings. One of the major problems encountered by the project was referring the drug users for an affordable drug treatment from the streets.

Conclusion

Since the late 1980, when HIV was first detected in India, very little attention has been given to its prevention among IDUs. Transmission of the virus through commercial sex workers and long-distance truck drivers was given more attention. HIV prevention activities among IDUs have been influenced by the existing legal system which does not allow distribution of injecting equipment to IDUs. The Narcotic Drug and Psychotropic Substance Abuse Act, which does not effectively differentiate between a drug user and someone who is involved in the trafficking of drugs, also influenced prevention activities among IDUs. In addition, the denial of the problem of HIV in general, and among IDUs as well, has contributed to the lack of interventions in the country.

Political denial and denial in the existing legal system have been manifested in the problems faced in implementing interventions in different cities. For example, in Manipur as well as in other states, the Narcotic Drug and Psychotropic Substance Abuse Act has been used to imprison users even though they have never been involved in trafficking or dealing in illicit drugs. In Manipur, more than 50 per cent of the drug users mentioned that they had been in prison at least once in their lives.

In Manipur and Kolkata, both the community and the local authorities were very much opposed to providing any risk-reduction measures, especially clean injecting equipment, to IDUs. Provision of bleach to clean injecting equipment as well as of sterile injecting equipment was seen as supporting drug use and not as measures for prevention of HIV. HIV/AIDS was perceived as a disease of the marginalised, such as prostitutes and those involved in immoral activities. It was never seen as a public health priority. It was not realised that preventing HIV among drug users would lead to preventing it among the larger community. Drug use was considered anti-social as well as immoral, and HIV/AIDS was considered to be a moral problem. Before implementing outreach targeting IDUs, outreach was conducted to the non-drug using community (marginalisation and discrimination of drug users and lack of services in general). It was vital to address the problems of marginalisation and discrimination as a first step in facilitating outreach to IDUs. The outreach to the larger community and advocacy among local leaders and law enforcement authorities helped implement interventions targeting IDUs.

The denial of the need to develop and implement interventions targeting IDUs has created many problems and obstacles. For both the state and local authorities, prevention of HIV among IDUs has not been a priority. This has been reflected in the activities developed and implemented by different agencies involved in drug abuse prevention, as they have not included HIV prevention among drug users. In Chennai, this was overcome largely by the formation of an umbrella organisation called Society for Prevention, Research and Education on Alcohol and Drugs. This helped in galvanising forces in HIV prevention efforts. A number of different organisations involved in drug abuse prevention also initiated HIV prevention activities in Chennai.

In Manipur, the intervention project generated a genuine interest in HIV prevention in the community. A number of HIV/AIDS prevention initiatives have been launched in Churachandpur and in other districts in the state. Three of the local NGOs have initiated small syringe-needle exchange programmes.

Even though HIV prevention activities targeting IDUs have been implemented in different parts of the country, a lot remains to be done. The virus is spreading faster than ever. The north-eastern states, especially Manipur, have high rates of HIV infection among IDUs. The project in Manipur was an intervention research study and was funded for three years, and ended in March 1997. However, it has been able to generate interests in HIV prevention among IDUs in the community. The success of the project depended on the attitude and beliefs of the larger community. This was gained through constant advocacy and outreach to the community. The project also helped in mobilising different groups in Manipur towards HIV prevention efforts. This was reflected in a request to the project staff made by the state authorities to establish syringe-needle exchange in Manipur.

The projects described in this chapter indicate the feasibility of establishing HIV prevention interventions targeting IDUs in the Indian setting. Even though outreach as a method of intervention was initiated in the United States and its feasibility not examined earlier in a developing country, the project in Manipur provided ample support that it was feasible to establish such interventions in India, and provide drug users with HIV/AIDS prevention information-education and risk-reduction materials.

Even though the syringe-needle exchanges established in Manipur have not yet been evaluated to examine their efficacy in changing risk behaviours among the IDUs in Manipur, it was, however, feasible to establish such interventions in India. The prevention activities initiated in Chennai provide testimony to the fact it was feasible to reach the IDUs, initiate risk reduction among them and develop consensus among other organisations in initiating HIV prevention activities.

Even though methadone maintenance has been accepted as one of the major treatment modalities in the United States and a number of other countries, the substitution method always generated controversy. The oral buprenrophine substitution project in Delhi has been successful in attracting a large number of injectors and providing them with HIV/AIDS prevention information-education. While methadone maintenance may not be cost effective in India, oral buprenrophine would be feasible for treating addiction and preventing HIV/AIDS.

Most of these interventions have been found to be effective in terms of implementation and in prevention of diseases. They were also found to be cost effective in reaching a large number of drug users and providing them with HIV/AIDS prevention information-education as well as risk-reduction materials. Given the current level of the epidemic and the extent of the spread of the virus, the interventions targeting IDUs need to be expanded throughout the country. It is important that the experiences learned from Manipur, Chennai, Kolkata and Delhi are replicated in other parts of the country and that similar interventions are implemented immediately.

International organisations and agencies have played a significant role in these projects, through providing some type of support. For example, the project in Manipur has been funded by the World Health Organization. The project in Delhi received funding from the European Commission. While the project in Chennai has not received direct support from international agencies, it has utilised findings from an assessment conducted in Chennai which was funded by WHO. The Kolkata project has not received any outside funding support. However, all the projects received some degree of technical support from different outside agencies and organisations outside.

The role of international agencies and organisations has been very significant and noteworthy. Given the lack of resources in the country, as well as the lack of political will to prevent HIV infection among drug users, the international agencies made it possible to implement interventions targeting IDUs. Support from international organisations also made it possible to generate political support from local and national authorities.

References/Further Reading

Abdul-Quader, A.S., D.C. Des Jarlais, S. Tross, et al., 1992. 'Outreach to Injecting Drug Users and Female Sexual Partners of Drug Users on the Lower East Side of New York City'. *British Journal of Addiction*, 87: 519–26.

Caplehorn, J.R. and **M.W. Ross,** 1995. 'Methadone Maintenance and the Likelihood of Risky Needle Sharing'. *International Journal of Addictions*, 30: 685–98.

Cartter, M.L., L.R. Petersen, R.B. Savage and **J. Donagher,** 1990. 'Providing HIV Counselling and Testing Services in Methadone Maintenance Programs'. *AIDS*, 4(5): 463–65.

Chatterjee, A., C.Z. Hangzo, A.S. Abdul-Quader, K.R. O'Reilly, G.T. Zomi and **S. Sarkar,** 1996. 'Evidence of Effectiveness of Street Based Outreach Intervention to Change Cleaning Behaviour among Injecting Drug Users in Manipur, India'. International Conference on AIDS, Vancouver.

Des Jarlais, D.C., G.V. Stimson, H. Hagan, D. Perlman, K. Choopanya, F.I. Bastos and **S.R. Friedman,** 1996. 'Emerging Infectious Diseases and the Injection of Illicit Psychoactive Drugs'. *Current Issues in Public Health,* 2: 102–37.

Des Jarlais, D.C., and **H. Maynard,** 1992. 'Evaluation of Needle Exchange Program on HIV Risk Behaviors'. Supplemented final report, AMFAR.

Des Jarlais, D.C., and **S.R. Friedman,** 1989. 'AIDS and IV Drug Use'. *Science,* 245: 578–79.

Dolan, K.A., G.V. Stimson and **M. Donoghoe,** 1993. 'Reductions in HIV Risk Behaviour and HIV Prevalence in Syringe-Exchange Clients and Other Injectors in England'. *Drug and Alcohol Review,* 12: 133–42.

Gleghorn, A.A., M.C. Doherty, D. Vlahov, D.D. Celentano and **T.S. Jones,** 1994. 'Inadequate Bleach Contact Times During Syringe Cleaning by Injection Drug Users'. *Journal of Acquired Immunodeficiency Syndromes,* 7: 762–72.

Hangzo, C.Z., A. Chatterjee, S. Sarkar, G.T. Zomi and **A.S. Abdul-Quader,** 1997. 'Reaching Out Beyond the Hills: HIV Prevention among the Injecting Drug Users in the North-Eastern State of Manipur'. *Addiction,* 92(7): 813–20.

Hartgers, C., E.C. Bunning, G.W. van Santen, A.D. Verster and **R.A. Coutinho,** 1989. 'The Impact of the Needle and Syringe-Exchange Programme in Amsterdam on Injecting Risk Behaviour. *AIDS,* 3: 571–76.

Higgins, D.L., C. Galavotti, K.R. O'Reilly, D.J. Schnell, M. Moore, D.L. Rugg, et al., 1991. 'Evidence for the Effects of HIV antibody Counselling and Testing on Risk Behaviours'. *Journal of the American Medical Association,* 266: 2419–29.

Indian Council of Medical Research, 1992–95. 'Unit for Research on AIDS in North-Eastern States of India'. Report. Calcutta.

————, 1996. 'Project on HIV/AIDS and Substance Abuse'. Annual Report.

Institute for Health Policy Studies, 1993. *The Public Health Impact of Needle Exchange Programs in the United States and Abroad: Summary, Conclusions and Recommendations.*

Kumar, S., W. Mandell, S.P. Thyagaraj, S. Solomon, Shakuntala Mudaliar and **D. Daniels,** 1995. 'HIV Risk Behavior of Injecting Buprenorphine Users in Madras City, India'. In program and abstracts of the 1995 Conference on AIDS and Drug Abuse, sponsored by NIDA and NIH in conjunction with 57th Annual Scientific Meeting, College of Problems of Drug Dependence.

Kumar, S. and **D. Daniels,** 1994. 'HIV Risk Reduction Strategies among IDUs in Madras: Assessment Research Report'.

Latkin, C., W. Mandell, M. Oziemkowska, D. Celentano, D. Vlahov, M. Ensminger and **A. Knowlton,** 1995. 'Using social network Analysis to Study Patterns of Drug Use among Urban Drug users at Risk for HIV/AIDS'. *Drugs and Alcohol Dependance,* 38: 1–9.

MMWR, 1993. 'Assessment of Street Outreach for HIV Prevention-Selected Sites, 1991–1993'. 19: 42(45): 873, 879–80.

Mudaliar, S. and **S. Kumar,** 1996. Comparative Analysis of HIV Sexual and Substance Use Risk Behaviors among Injecting Heroin Users and Buprenorphine Users in a Drug Treatment Program. In *Abstracts of Building International Research in Drug Abuse: Opportunites and Challenges.* Sponsored by NIDA in conjunction with the 58th Annual Scientific Meeting, College on Problems of Drug Dependence.

Neaigus, A., M. Sufian, S.R. Friedman, et al., 1990. 'Effects of Outreach Intervention on Risk Reduction among Intravenous Drug Users'. *AIDS Education and Prevention*, 2: 253–71.

National Institute of Health, 1997. NIH Consensus Statement. Interventions to Prevent HIV Risk Behaviours. 15(2).

Ostrow, D.G., 1989. 'AIDS Prevention through Effective Education'. *Daedalus*, 118: 229–54.

Panda, S. and A. Chatterjee, 1997. 'A Mid-term Evaluation of "Drug Demand Reduction Project for Delhi Slums"'. *SHARAN*.

Panda, S., A. Chatterjee, S. Bhattacharjee, B. Ray, M.K. Saha and S.K. Bhattacharya, 1998. 'HIV, Hepatitis B and Sexual Practices in the Street Recruited Injecting Drug Users of Calcutta: Risk Perception Versus Observed Risks'. *International Journal of STD and AIDS*, 9(4): 214–18.

Panda, S., A. Chatterjee, S. Sarkar, K.N. Jalan, T. Maitra, S. Mukherjee, et al., 1997. 'Injection Drug Use in Calcutta: A Potential Focus for an Explosive HIV Epidemic'. *Drug and Alcohol Review*, 16: 17–23.

Panda, S., T. Nabachandra, S. Sarkar, S. Chakraborty, T.N. Naik and B.C. Deb, 1994. 'Herpes Zoster in an HIV-positive 14-month-old baby'. *The National Medical Journal of India*, 7(2): 63–64.

Sarkar, S., S. Panda, K. Sarkar, C.Z. Hangzo, L. Bijaya, N.Y. Singh, A. Agarwal, A. Chatterjee, B.C. Deb and R. Detels, 1995. 'A Cross-Sectional Study on Factors Determining Unsafe Injecting Practices Including HIV Testing and Counselling among Injecting Drug Users of Manipur'. *Indian Journal of Public Health*, 39(3): 86–92.

Stimson, G.V., 1989. 'Syringe-Exchange Programmes for Injecting Drug Users: Editorial Review'. *AIDS*, 3: 253–60.

Titus, S., M. Marmor, D.C. Des Jarlais, M. Kim, H. Wolfe and S. Beatrice, 1994. 'Bleach Use and HIV Seroconversion among New York City Injection Drug Users'. *Journal of Acquired Immunodeficiency Syndromes*, 7: 700–704.

Vlahov, D., J. Astemborski, L. Solomon and K.E. Nelson, 1994. 'Field Effectiveness of Needle Disinfection among Injecting Drug Users'. *Journal of the Acquired Immunodeficiency Syndromes*, 7: 760–66.

Weibel, W., A. Jimenez, W. Johnson, L. Ouellet, T. Lampinen, J. Murray, et al., 1993. 'Positive Effect on HIV Seroconversion of Street Outreach Intervention with IDU in Chicago: 1988–1992'. Abstract No. WS-C15-2. IXth International Conference on AIDS, Berlin, 1993.

8

Female Commercial Sex Workers: An Innovative Intervention from West Bengal

Smarajit Jana, Suparna Ghosh, Debashis Bose, Sanchita Chowdhury and *Kamala Mukherjee*

Initiation

The first case of HIV in India was detected in Chennai in the year 1986. In the same year, a full-blown case of AIDS was reported from another metropolis in the country (NACO 1996). Professional blood donors, intravenous drug users and antenatal mothers run the risk of getting infected with the virus but, the heterosexual mode of transmission being the predominant one, commercial sex workers (CSWs) are at highest risk. Recognising the link between commercial sex work and HIV transmission, the Government of India has given high priority to HIV prevention among commercial sex workers and their clients in its national plan.

As a part of this strategy, an STD (sexually transmitted disease)/HIV intervention programme was launched in Sonagachi, one of the oldest and largest red-light districts in the city of Kolkata. It is estimated that about 4,000 active CSWs reside in nearly 370 brothels in this locality, with a seasonal variation of upto 1000. Except in the peak season, from September to October, a floating population of around 1,500 sex workers may also be found in the vicinity throughout the year.

The intervention project, which was initiated in September 1992 with support from the NACO (National AIDS Control Organisation) and the WHO (World Health Organization) and subsequently from NORAD (Norwegian Royal Embassy for Development) and finally from ODA (Overseas Development Administration; now known as Department for International Development), was based on a random sample STD survey conducted from May to June 1992—the first such study carried out in India. This baseline survey was conducted by AIIH & PH (All India Institute of Hygiene & Public Health) in collaboration with local NGOs (non-governmental organisations) and CBOs (community-based organisations). It looked at the social demography of the locality, mapped the sexual practices among the CSWs and their clients and partners, and assessed the prevalence of STDs and HIV among them.

About 12 per cent of the sex workers living in the locality were surveyed and the following socio-demographic aspects were highlighted—85 per cent of the sex workers surveyed were between the ages of 15 and 29 years, literacy rates among those surveyed were very low and alcohol abuse was common. Poverty was cited as the dominant reason for entering into the sex trade. Of the 450 sex workers surveyed, 40 per cent had children, 45 per cent used contraception in some form and only 27 per cent used it regularly. Only 2.7 per cent used condoms always or often, 69 per cent had knowledge of STDs and 31 per cent had heard of AIDS. Laboratory results revealed that five out of the 442 serum samples surveyed tested positive for HIV infection, the positivity rate being 1.1 per cent (Jana et al. 1998).

Objectives

The project had three principal components—provision of health services, including STD treatment; information, education and communication; and condom programming. The objectives of the project were:

- to reduce the incidence of STD/HIV infection among the sex workers and their clients in the target area through adequate provision of health services

- to develop and implement appropriate laboratory support services for STD case management
- to provide an entry point to CSWs for education and awareness-raising activities and for condom promotion among the target group
- to maintain and expand the relationship of trust and confidence established between the implementors of the project and the community in order to generate support for AIDS prevention programmes
- to increase the awareness of STDs and HIV/AIDS among the sex workers, madams, pimps and clients
- to motivate the sex workers and their clients to use condoms for each sexual encounter
- to develop generic guidelines for the progression of intervention programmes, which could be replicated in similar areas.

Methodology Adopted

The concept of peer educators was introduced to establish a link between members of the target community and the project staff. This concept recognises sex workers as a professional group, inculcates confidence in them, enhances their self esteem, and empowers and encourages them to take an active part in the project activities. Peer educators are recruited from among the CSWs. They are required to take a six-week training programme on STDs and HIV comprising classroom teaching and field-based orientations on the issues of HIV/AIDS, and have to pass an oral test as well (Fox 1994). The peer educators spend a part of their working day distributing condoms, spreading awareness about STDs and motivating sex workers to attend the STD clinics. The more experienced peer educators get involved in training new peer educators and other community members.

Growth

The basic approach of the project was based on three R's—respect, reliance and recognition. Respect of sex workers, recognising their work as a profession and relying on their understanding were crucial factors when programme activities were designed and implemented. Being a process, the project encouraged experimentation, selecting activities and modifying strategies in accordance with the requirements of the field reality.

In 1992, a health service centre was opened on the premises of a local youth club in Sonagachi which was attended by sex workers and members of their family. The clinic emphasises diagnosis and treatment of STDs and follows the syndrome-based management approach. It also caters to general health requirements of sex workers and their children. An evening clinic which mainly caters to the clients of sex workers was also initiated in Sonagachi (Jana and Banerjee 1997). Encouraged by the number of sex workers who visited the clinic and the demand for quality medicare services, health service centres were successively opened in 10 other red-light areas in the city—Rambagan, Sethbagan, Bowbazar, Kalighat, Tollygunj, Lakharmath, Wattgunj, Chetla, Ghoradana and Bandhaghat.

The startegy of STD management as planned in the original proposal was very much dependent on laboratory investigations. Treatment was to be based on the traditional approach of etiopathological diagnosis of STD cases. It was soon realised that this approach could not ensure the quality of STD care services, that it delayed the institution of treatment and besides, that there was a lack of quality laboratory facilities. So, the project shifted from etiopathological diagnosis of STD cases to syndromic case management although this was also not a foolproof strategy. Later, to tackle the high prevalence of syphilis, opportunistic screening of syphilis through the VDRL (venereal disease research laboratory) test was introduced.

Development

In the course of these activities, the peer group of workers started to realise the grim reality of their trade and profession and the lack of power to gain control over their sexual practices. They gradually felt the necessity of improving their standard of living and excercising control, not only over sexual practices in order to ensure safety, but over many other relevant issues in relation to their families, their babus (permanent partners of sex workers who maintain a husband-like relationship) and clients. The project helped the sex workers realise the need for effectively articulating demands, enhancing negotiation skills, securing a stable income, the availability of proper living conditions and the proper rearing of their siblings. Thus they came up with their own articulated demands for activities such as non-formal education, self-banking system and the formation of a cultural forum.

How the Demands were Created

Non-formal Education

A Case Study   One day, a peer educator complained that they had to keep accounts, write short reports and applications for leave, read various published materials, etc., and only a small section of them, who had had initial schooling, proved competent at this while the lack of literacy created a regular problem for the others. The peer educators expressed their desire to learn to read and write. This urge for literacy emanated from their will to become more effective workers (Jana and Banerjee 1997).

A non-formal system of learning was developed as a product of participatory interaction with a focus on the sex workers' mental and physical well being, which was also appropriate for their age and environment. The prime aim of the system was to build up a meaningful learning process for the specific group of women so that in the course of learning to read and write they may also learn to reflect upon themselves and redefine their role in society.

When the education programme began in Sonagachi, in 1992, it catered to only 12 students (peer educators). The number has since gone up to 247 and the programme has been extended to eight other centres. The programme initially imparted basic reading and some writing skills to the sex workers and from this phase, 35 students were selected for the advanced non-formal education programme called Digangana. This phase of the programme was designed to cover areas such as health, language and communication. The programme did not follow a rigid structure and the learners also offered a lot of suggestions to enrich the programme.

In collaboration with other NGOs, an education programme for the children of sex workers also started at the red-light areas of Rambagan and Sethbagan in 2000, and it is attended by about 573 children.

Usha Cooperative

A Case Study   One day, a sex worker from Sonagachi said that there was a decline in the market and that clients were not pouring in as they used to. She said that she, like other sex workers, would have to borrow money from the moneylender at exorbitant rates of interest and would again land in an acute financial crisis. She added that for every loan of Rs 500, they would have to pay Rs 10 a day as interest. By the time they finally managed to repay the loan (within two months and 12 days as per the condition), the total amount they would each have paid would be Rs 1,200. The sex workers badly wanted to escape the clutches of these moneylenders.

Thus the idea of a cooperative run by sex workers took shape in 1995 and it was called Usha Multipurpose Co-operative Society Ltd. This cooperative caters exclusively to the sex workers and was registered under the West Bengal Co-operative Societies Act, 1983. It started with 13 members and now has 3,528 members; it acts as a credit cooperative and provides loans to its members at reasonable rates of interest. Basanti Sena, a group of sex workers, selected and trained by the cooperative to market, promote and sell condoms, carries out social marketing of condoms in 45 red-light areas in different parts of West Bengal. Through social marketing, the cooperative has been able to generate good business and extensive demand for condoms. The cooperative also runs an evening/night creche for the children of sex workers. Future plans of the cooperative include running a department store with items of daily use, establishing a vocational training unit and a production unit of jute handicraft, setting up a small pathology laboratory for some routine diagnoses, and initiating development activities for sex workers and their families through recycling funds.

The Formation of a Sex Workers' Forum

A Case Study   One day, a peer educator said that the sex workers has been thinking of forming an action committee for quite some time because they felt that the project should not get involved in every local hassle that comes up and that the sex workers should unite through networking, tackle their problems on their own and themselves fight all the injustice done to them, particularly by law enforcement personnel. With a view to creating a platform to do this, the Durbar Mahila Samanwaya Committee (DMSC), a forum of sex workers, was formed. Presently it has a membership of over 65,000 sex workers, representing different red-light areas of West Bengal, and 62 branches spread out through the state. DMSC, in an attempt to change the society's view towards women engaged in the sex trade, had undertaken several activities, a few of which are listed here.

(a) Programmes or measures undertaken to ensure the safety of sex workers and their children in different red-light areas
   (i) Whenever the police conducts large-scale raids in red-light areas, DMSC members get together and protest against this persecution by conducting rallies.
   (ii) An NGO in central Kolkata experimented with an unqualified AIDS vaccine on hapless sex workers without taking their consent, which was vehemently opposed by DMSC.
   (iii) DMSC protested against the inhuman beating up of children of some sex workers kept at a non-government home in Barasat.
   (iv) On 12 September 1998 sex workers (SWs) participated in a rally organised against the illegal and inhuman attempts of eviction of SWs from the Rampurhat lane in the Babubazar area of Khiderpur in South Kolkata.
   (v) On 3 August 1999 DMSC gheraoed the office of the Bangladesh High Commission in Kolkata protesting against the eviction of sex workers in Tanbazar.
   (vi) On 10 October 2000 DMSC organised a rally against eviction of Bashirhat red-light area.
(b) Programmes organised to improve the working and living conditions of sex workers and their families.
   (i) A centre for counselling and social support was opened in 1996 at Rambagan, a red-light area in the city, to provide counselling in connection to personal, familial and any other problems of sex workers, and also other support services.

(ii) DMSC has launched various programmes to prevent the entry of female minors in the sex trade.

(iii) The organisation has successfully conducted national conferences of sex workers at Kolkata which have been attended by thousands of sex workers from all over the country and from abroad.

The Formation of Komal Gandhar

During the various activities of DMSC, it was observed that sex workers had an immense cultural potential and, if provided with an adequate forum of expression, this potential could be utilised as an educational tool, more so in the context of a community with low literacy rates, and also as an effective medium of communication facilitating self-expression and self-identity.

Thus was Komal Gandhar, the cultural wing of DMSC, formed. At present it has 79 members including female and male sex workers and their children. The members express themselves through various cultural activities such as music, dance, drama, painting and writing, to promote the message 'Making Sex Work Safe'. This forum provides sex workers and their children an opportunity to bring their dormant talents. Komal Gandhar participated in the inaugural ceremony and the cultural programmes at the 12th World AIDS Conference held in Geneva. The troupe also presented a play at the 14th National Theatre Festival in Kolkata in collaboration with Nandikar, a renowned theatre group of the city. Through street plays and group songs, Komal Gandhar also promotes the social marketing of condoms.

Positive Hotline

One day, a peer educator came to one of the doctors in the clinic and reported that she had heard of an AIDS patient in Burdwan. The patient and her family were not being allowed by the other villagers to buy food from the local shops or use the local pond. Thus was born in the minds of the project staff a need to respond to the problem of HIV+ people.

The project started operating an HIV helpline called Positive Hotline, which is the first telephone hotline for HIV+ and seropositive people and AIDS patients and their families in the state of West Bengal. This HIV helpline was inaugurated on 28 November 1996 by Smt. Minati Ghosh, then Minister of Family Welfare, Government of West Bengal. Personnel for Positive Hotline comprises a group of volunteers including doctors, nurses, counsellors and legal experts. Upon receiving a telephone call, this group visits the caller at home or at any place suited to the caller and, through advocacy, counselling and providing information on medical assistance and legal aid, helps the patient and the family cope with the trauma associated with being HIV+.

Problems Faced

The entire sex trade scenario is controlled by a landlord–politician–police nexus dominated by local mafias, and the sex workers are on the lowest rung of this power structure. Social unacceptance of the profession, gender inequality, low socio-economic status of the sex workers reflected in their lack of power to control their professional activities, get information about safer sexual practices, overcome inhuman working conditions and have rights over their bodies, present almost insurmountable hurdles to behaviour change. As the practices of safer sex cannot be dealt with in isolation, the project adopted the strategy of the empowerment of sex workers. Thus, a number of varied activities unrelated to AIDS became a part of the project as the perceptive needs of the community were given priority.

The services delivered by the project involved the members of the target community in carrying out various activities for their well being. This had an impact over the different power groups controlling the sex trade, and certain problems started to evolve. Since the project staff insisted on consistent condom use, the madams apprehended a loss in their income. Local clubs that used to extract money from the sex workers on some pretext or the other feared that the empowerment of sex workers would minimise their contol over the sex workers.

Conflicts were palpable at different levels during the implementation of the project. Although the government considers the services rendered by the project as a pro-people activity, several high officials belonging to the class of 'policy-makers' started criticising the programme, raising the issue of morality. They claimed that the project was promoting immoral practices and 'pampering' sex workers.

NGOs with abolitionist policies who work with sex worker communities generally prescribe rehabilitation as the only way of their upliftment and question the newer strategy of empowering sex workers.

The activities undertaken by the project staff made researchers feel threatened as the sex worker community used to act as the 'object' of research activities and, in many circumstances, they even dared to flout ethical guidelines. They felt uncomfortable to see the changes in terms of the empowerment of the sex workers. The research groups objected to the strategy of intervention which upheld human dignity and self-esteem and considered it superfluous and redundant for intervention. They wanted the project staff to go back to prototypical condom promotion and STD awareness.

Advocacy and liaisoning with the government, with NGOs and with the different stakeholders of this trade, eased these problems to a considerable extent. Also, the target community had to be convinced that the project would not interfere with the sex trade.

Success

With the development of these activities, appreciable changes in sexual practices could be achieved that were reflected in increased condom use and steady reduction in STDs. By 1994–95, when the project received remarkable national and international acclaim for these achievements, the sex worker community was greatly impressed. The appreciated the success of the project in:

- generating a sense of self-respect, social identity and recognition
- providing multi-faceted scopes for the development of aptitude and skills in different spheres of social activities
- improving communication and better negotiation between sex workers and other members of community and between sex workers and different power-holders operating within the sex trade
- facilitating the expression of sex workers' felt needs and developing a professional attitude with a sense of social responsibility

- facilitating individual and organised resistance against various oppressions and exploitations creating a platform for sex workers and networking among sex workers for integration and solidarity.

These perceived successes were expressed in focus group discussions with the sex workers.

Sampling Techniques Undertaken During Surveys for Evaluation

During the first random sample STD survey carried out in 1992, multistage sampling was undertaken to obtain proper representation. A census was made by the survey team to prepare a list of premises, the number of brothels and number of sex workers in each brothel. They identified 362 brothels, where 3,664 sex workers resided. The sex workers were stratified into three categories according to their professional charges, access to water and sanitation facilities and possesion of assets such as electric fan, radio, television and furniture. Sex workers who changed more than Rs 100 per client were included in category A, those who charged between Rs 50 and Rs 100 per client were included in category B and those who charged less than Rs 50 per client fell in category C. Apart from brothel-based sex workers, there were many 'floating' sex workers who would rent a room for a short period, entertain clients and vacate the room. As it was not possible to establish their number, they were excluded from the survey. A few sex workers who used to work independently (self-employed) were also excluded from the first survey. There were 724 sex workers in category A, 1,772 in category B and 1,168 sex workers in category C. A brothel was taken as a unit of sample and 65 brothels were randomly selected. Of these 12 were in category A, 28 in category B and 25 in category C. The number of sex workers selected from each category was proportional to the total number of sex workers in each stratum. Usually, six or seven sex workers were randomly selected from each of the 65 brothels. If the number of sex workers in a brothel was less then the size required, some were selected from the next brothel to cover the deficit. Replacement for 'non-responders', or absentees, was also found from the next brothels. Thus, 81, 209 and 160 sex workers were selected from categories A, B and C respectively. The total number of sex workers surveyed was 450.

Table 8.1

HIV prevalence in four consecutive surveys among
female sex workers at Sonagachi

Year	Tested*	HIV-+ve (%)	95% CI
1992	442	05 (1.13)	0.15–2.11%
1993	607	07 (1.15)	0.30–2.11%
1995	582	28 (4.81)	3.07–6.55%
1998	506	28 (5.53)	3.54–7.52%

CI= Confidence Interval

*In 1992 and 1993, 450 and 612 samples were collected respectively, and 442 and 607 of these could be tested; the reasons being breakage of vials and haemolysis of blood during transport. In 1995 and 1998, the sample size was increased to 590 and 510 respectively, to have a better idea of HIV prevalence among sex workers. The samples tested were 582 and 506, which were again less than those collected, for the same reasons cited here.

In order to assess the effectiveness and impact of the project, repeated cross-sectional surveys (see Table 8.1) were carried out by the project team. During these subsequent surveys that were carried out in 1993, 1995 and 1998, the basic parameters of the previous multistage sampling were followed with minor variations, keeping in view the changing scenario of the sex trade. In the first repeat survey of 1993, 612 sex workers were studied by random sampling. In the second and third, self-employed sex workers were also included as a unit of sampling. Five hundred and ninety sex workers were studied in the survey of 1995 and 510 in the survey of 1998.

Data for survey was collected by interview, physical examination and laboratory testing. One of the indicators considered in the successive surveys was increased practice of condom use by the clients of sex workers, which was judged through self-addressed questionnaires. Declining rates of STD infection and seropositivity were also considered important indicators of behaviour change in these repeat surveys.

While analysing condom use by the clients of sex workers (see Table 8.2), it was observed that even sex workers coming to the red-light areas for a very short span of time, some for a period as short as less than three months, were able to convince their clients to use condoms. This fact highlights an important issue of intervention strategy—that it is peer pressure and not mere education about safer sexual practices that helps in active motivation for condom use.

Table 8.2
Percentage of sex workers using condoms

Survey	Number of respondents	Always (%)	Often (%)
1992 (Apr.–May)	450	1.1	1.6
1993 (Nov.–Dec.)	612	47.2	22.1
1995 (Aug.–Sep.)	590	50.1	31.6
1998 (Apr.–May)	510	50.4	40.1

Table 8.3
Results of serological tests for syphillis (VDRL positivity in 1:8
and above dilution) in four consecutive surveys

Year	Tested	VDRL positivity (%)	95% CI
1992	417	25.42	(21.24%–29.60%)
1993	607	28.5	(24.91%–32.09%)
1995	475	14.1	(10.97%–17.23%)
1998	506	11.46	(8.68%–14.23%)

CI = Confidence Interval

The formation of the forum of sex workers helped them to unite and carry out various development activities. This forum carried out networking in the different red-light areas with the mission of unifying sex workers under a common banner. Networking also instilled self-respect and confidence among the sex workers, not only at individual levels but also at the social level. It helped sex workers muster political power and the will to communicate to different sections of the society, including in the negotiation of safer sexual practices with clients. Through the cooperative, the sex workers could avail loan at reasonable rates of interest, which helped to reduce their economic vulnerability and provided a support base for the betterment of their living and working conditions. Provision of quality medicare services helped in the reduction of STD cases and HIV transmission.

There is a strong correlation between consistency of condom use and VDRL seropositivity as observed from Tables 8.3 and 8.4. This shows that the prevention component of the intervention programme achieved a reduction in STDs in this high-risk group. Also, it may be one of the reasons for the slow rise of HIV in this group.

Table 8.4
Distribution of condom use among CSWs (all categories)
vs. VDRL Reactiveness

	Condom Practice*			
	Always	Often	Sometimes	Never
VDRL (+ve)	37	75	18	5
% (+ve)	14.51	36.95	45	62.50
(95% CI)	(10.19%– 18.83%)	(30.31%– 43.59%)	(29.59%– 60.41%)	(28.95%– 96.05%)
VDRL (–ve)	218	128	22	3
% (–ve)	85.49	63.05	55	7.50
(95% CI)	(81.17%– 89.81%)	(56.41%– 69.69%)	(39.59%– 70.41%)	(3.95%– 71.05%)

CI = Confidence Interval

*Of the 506 sex workers surveyed in 1998, it was found that the number who always used condoms was 255; often used condoms—203; sometimes used condoms—40; and the number who never used condoms was eight.

Hurdles

(i) Attempts made in the red-light areas to reach the clients of sex workers have not so far produced very encouraging results.

(ii) During the education classes that were conducted for the sex workers, it was generally observed that there is a decline in retention ability of old sex workers for the lessons taught. A lack of sustained interest is another major impediment to adult learning. In the context of non-formal education of sex workers, the problem is compounded by the non-availability of learning time, by community squabbles, economic anxieties, etc.

(iii) The project felt the need for addressing the entire section of floating population of sex workers in the area, a group that is very difficult to target because of its migratory nature. Unless awareness of STDs/HIV is reached to this particular group, condom usage promoted among them and health care services made available to them, it is very difficult to contain the spread of STDs/HIV.

(iv) Unsafe sexual practices by the local babus, who ensnare sex workers in a web of infatuation and passion and convince them to engage in sexual practices without condoms, are difficult to motivate. This results in repeated infection of sex workers.

(v) Pimps have a grip over sex workers of all categories. It so happens at times that sex workers reluctantly accept a diseased client due to pressure from the pimps.

(vi) Due to the stigma attached to the profession and lack of awareness of proper treatment for STDs, the sex workers prefer to go to quacks and resort to other locally prevalent unscientific methods of treatment. Consequently, they are mistreated or half treated and their problems are compounded.

Sustainability

The ultimate target of the project is the self-sufficiency of the sex worker community. Ample food, suitable housing, satisfactory educational opportunities, adequate health care and occupational prospects will determine the level of self-sufficiency. All these have been planned to be achieved through different activities that help sustainability at different levels.

Social Sustainability

The project aims at enhancing self-esteem and a positive attitude among the community members so that they show an active interest, involvement and responsibility, resulting in the amalgamation and perpetuation of the project activities. Ownership of the various development programmes is a criterion for sustainability which is possible through an attitude of responsibility and liability in the community and a participatory approach to decision-making. Training programmes, workshops, seminars and exposure visits help in the capacity-building of the sex workers, which serves as a foundation for economic sustainability.

Economic Sustainability

• Local resources can be mobilised in various ways for the interests of the community.

- The members of the sex workers' organisation contribute a monthly membership fee which is utilised for various community development activities.
- Through social marketing of condoms, the dual purpose of making quality condoms available at affordable prices to sex workers and profit generation is served. The profit is used to sustain project activities.
- The sex workers and their children who visit the clinic are charged a nominal fee, which is utilised in providing quality medicare services.

Conclusion

The most important lesson learnt from the project is that it is not enough to design a technically sound and efficient intervention programme to improve the health status of sex workers and control STD/HIV infection among them. The introduction of intervention components in response to the perceived needs of the community to evolve a comprehensive development programme, the active participation of sex workers at all levels, including policy-making, transparent management, democratic functioning, readjustment with power lobbies, reduction in the gap between the interests of project and the common interests of the sex workers, are some of the key elements that need to be incorporated into the project planning. This kind of approach broadens the sphere from a narrow STD/HIV intervention programme to a sexual health programme which in the future might develop into a community-based programme of sex workers, for sex workers and by sex workers.

References/Further Reading

Fox, Robin, 1994. 'Red Light on Calcutta; Health via School in Andhra Pradesh'. *Lancet*, October, p. 4.

Jana, Smarajit and Bhaskar Banerjee (eds) 1997. 'Seven Years' Stint'. Report prepared by Sanchita Chowdhury and Nandinee Banerjee.

Jana, Smarajit, Nandinee Bandopadhayay, Sadhana Mukherjee, Nayanita Dutta, Ishika Basu and Amitrajit Saha, 1998. 'STD/HIV Intervention with Sex Workers in W. Bengal, India'. *AIDS*, vol. 12, suppl. B, p. 3.

National AIDS Control Organisation (NACO), 1996. 'Monthly Update on HIV Infection in India'. New Delhi: Ministry of Health and Family Welfare, p. 1.

HIV and Law in India

Subhram Rajkhowa

Introduction

AIDS has become a serious health concern the world over. It has been affecting the adult population disproportionately and millions of children have lost one or both parents to this pandemic. Of the estimated 3.86 million HIV-infected people in India, women and children constitute a sizable majority (NACO 2000). Moreover, 50 per cent of the infected population belongs to the age group of 15 to 24 years (UNAIDS/WHO 1998).

The situation in India is very alarming, with HIV spreading quickly across the country. According to the 1998 UNAIDS report, the HIV-infection rate in India at under 1 per cent of the total adult population, though considered low by the standards of many countries, is over 10 times higher than the rate in neighbouring China. The 3.86 million infections makes India the country with the second-largest number of HIV-infected people in the world. The lack of knowledge among the common people and their inability to protect themselves due to the lack of an adequate support system had led many an unfortunate victim of HIV/AIDS to suffer a lot of discrimination at the hands of medical and paramedical staff, and also from the society in general. The law has an important role in complementing and assisting education and other public health measures to generate awareness. Legislation needs to provide for non-discrimination and privacy so as to facilitate full community participation and the integration of HIV+ people in society by securing their trust and cooperation, and not compound the stigmatisation and alienation of this group of people, whom the society has rejected, by treating them in a negative, punitive way.

HIV Legislation

It is important to realise that, unlike the virus, discrimination and breaches of privacy are created by society, just as law to 'limit man's inhumanity to man' can be (Watchers 1995). The need for legislation cannot be underestimated although its drafting may be complex. Complexities may arise, for instance, due to inherent contradictions necessitating exceptions. It is precisely due to this reason that the drafting of AIDS legislation to meet the needs of the infected and the affected should be done with great care. In order to provide for a comprehensive legislation, foreign models also need to be considered. One cannot ignore the fact that the general principles of AIDS legislation are universally applicable. According to Watcher (1995), AIDS law should not be seen as a Western luxury by the developing world but as a basic human system which can be cheaply enacted and adequately enforced.

As of now, the enforcement mechanism is expensive and it therefore has to be adapted to suit local situation. Legislation has to be effective and not self-defeating by driving people who are at risk of or with the infection underground. A comprehensive policy to minimise the impact of HIV/AIDS is required, wherein the guidelines of WHO, UNAIDS and the Commission on Human Rights should be incorporated to the maximum extent. Such legislation, while providing for confidentiality, should at the same time be non-discriminatory in accordance with the United Nations Resolution No. 1995/44 passed by the Commission on Human Rights. This resolution calls upon states to 'ensure where necessary that the laws, policies and practices, including those in the context of HIV/AIDS respect human rights standards, including the right to privacy and integrity of people living with HIV/AIDS, prohibit HIV/AIDS related discrimination and do not have the effect of inhibiting programmes for prevention of HIV/AIDS and for the care of persons infected with HIV/AIDS'.

These concerns have become all the more serious over the years as AIDS has sharpened the focus on related legal, ethical and human rights issues that permeate all efforts to deal with the indivisibly growing pandemic in a more practical and humane manner. It raises many pertinent issues, including mandatory testing, discriminatory practices in employment and other ethical and moral counters as well. Comprehensive legislation incorporating prevention and control have been enacted in over one hundred countries. These include the Asian countries of China, Indonesia, Japan, Mongolia and Vietnam. It may be observed that there has been some progress on the legislative front in various parts of the globe, but the same has not been the case with India. Apart from Goa, which has a local statute and employs provisions of the Drugs and Cosmetics Act, 1940, the existing legislation in India with respect to communicable diseases is not adequate to deal with HIV/AIDS.

Human Rights and the Public Health Policy

A multipronged approach to the problem in consonance with human rights obligations is called for as human rights provide a critical perspective in the evaluation of AIDS policies. Therefore, legal mechanisms need to reflect the basic rights of individuals in accordance with the various international charters and declarations. But any legislation in this regard should first consider whether, in the interest of humanity at large, it should adopt an isolationist or an integrationist approach. For, in contrast to the isolationist approach, the integrationist approach does not require mandatory testing, but informed consent. It also provides for both pre- and post-test counselling, maintaining confidentiality of HIV status, besides providing for dignity through anti-discriminatory treatment. Such an approach is also in consonance with the Universal Declaration of Human Rights as well as the European Charter of Human Rights. Even the World Health Organization advocates the latter approach as it treats the patient as central to the strategy to combat the spread HIV/AIDS (Grover 1993).

The Commission on Human Rights Resolution No. 1994/49 also calls upon states to take all necessary steps, including appropriate and speedy redressal proceedings, to ensure the full enjoyment of civil, economic, social and cultural rights by people with HIV/AIDS, besides urging upon states to review their legislation and practices to ensure the right to privacy and integrity of persons with HIV/AIDS and those presumed to be at risk of infection. The following year (in Resolution No. 1995/44) it further called upon states to ensure that their laws, policies and practices including the right to privacy prohibit HIV-related discrimination. Recently, the Commission on Human Rights in its 57th meeting (1997/33) issued a number of guidelines, the third of which observed that 'states should review and reform public health law to ensure that they adequately address public health issues raised by HIV/AIDS, that their provisions applicable to casually transmitted diseases are not inappropriately applied to HIV/AIDS and that they are consistent with international human rights obligations'. Similarly, the fourth guideline re-emphasises the review and reform of criminal laws and correctional systems to ensure that they are not abused or misused in the context of HIV/AIDS or targeted against vulnerable groups. Guideline five calls upon the states to enact or strengthen anti-discrimination and other protective laws to remove discrimination and ensure privacy and confidentiality and ethics, apart from providing effective civil and administrative remedies.

Non-discrimination

Discrimination has been a major issue in the field of HIV/AIDS as affected individuals continue to be discriminated against, resulting in their victimisation. Discriminatory treatment continues to be meted out to affected individuals despite established and uncontroverted evidence that HIV/AIDS cannot be contacted by casual contact. Issues of summary dismissal of workers, debarring of children from attending schools, refusal of insurance companies to provide health insurance, and the like, are heard of even today in India as well as in other countries. Discrimination is exercised in the form restrictions imposed on the free movement of infected individuals. At times, quarantine or isolation, and compulsory hospitalisation have been taken recourse to. Such practices continue to be exercised because of prejudice and misinformation or the lack of information. There is a perceptible increase in the number of HIV-infected people in India being traumatised at the workplace due peer rejection and hostility from employers, even leading to outright dismissal (Mallikarjun 1998).

Discrimination in Education

A large segment of people affected by HIV/AIDS is in the age group of 15 to 24 years. Many of them, being students, have had their problems further compounded by the denial of educational facilities in some form or the other. In many other countries, parents of such students have sued boards and authorities of state-managed educational institutions for denial of admissions or for providing home-bound institutions. Such students have sometimes been singled out through placement in separate 'modular' classrooms, being accompanied by adults in field trips. In the mid-1980s they were discriminated to such an extent that some instances of isolation inside glass booths placed in a corner of the class were also reported (Lawyers Collective 1998).

While in most of the cases the courts have held prohibition of HIV+ students from attending schools as a retrograde step and directed their admission without segregation, in certain others the courts have directed the adoption of awareness programmes as well. They have gone to the extent of directing the introduction of sexual and drug addiction counselling for students, parents and the entire school system (Report on Discrimination 1983–87). Since HIV/AIDS cannot be spread through casual contact, the law should provide that no discrimination whatsoever shall be permitted in any institution offering general or technical education.

Discrimination in Employment

Discrimination at the workplace is another important issue deserving legal attention. In extreme cases if an HIV+ person happens to be terminated from service, not only does the person lose the prospect of future employment, the very existence of the person's family is at stake. Since HIV infection is not a cause for termination of employment, persons with HIV-related illnesses should be allowed to work as long as they are medically fit. The right to work of an HIV-infected person not only includes the right to equal opportunity of employment, but security of tenure, common and favourable conditions of work, the right to form and join trade unions and workers' organisations as well. It is important to understand that the right also includes freedom against all forms of discrimination in the workplace without having to undergo any mandatory HIV testing, without being under the fear of demotion, transfer or harassment in any form from his co-employees; not to speak of resignation or forced termination. In other words, employers cannot choose to discriminate against workers with HIV/AIDS and in the event of any such discrimination they should be entitled to adequate legal redress. The purpose of law is to ensure non discriminatory treatment through supportive legislation. It has to ensure community participation and integration of people living with HIV/AIDS at the workplace through trust and cooperation. Legislative enactment should lead to elimination of discrimination and any possible stigmatisation.

India in the Process of Finding Ways

The AIDS epidemic in India deserves serious attention by both the government and the society. Apart from concrete measures on the health front and the need for awareness programmes, legislation is required not only to supplement and complement the other measures, but also to minimise the risk of the further spread of the infection by safeguarding the rights of people infected with HIV, as well as people vulnerable to infection.

It is unfortunate that no legislative measures have yet been adopted in the statute books, apart from the Goa Act. This Act too has come in for a lot of criticism. It has many lacunae and, therefore, cannot be considered a guiding light for other states to follow. The isolation of HIV+ people is the premise of this law. Clause VII of Section 53(i) of the Act makes it mandatory for a person to be isolated if found positive to serological tests. Similarly, a reading of clauses VII, X and XII clearly establishes that the Act considers HIV/AIDS a contagious disease. Unfortunately, the Act passed legal scrutiny on being challenged in the Bombay High Court. Because of a strong belief that the Act is unjust and in violation of Constitutional principles, it was amended in 1989, doing away with the mandatory character of clause VII. Yet, the Act has been charged with not being in conformity with the principle of the right to equality as provided for under Article 14 of the Constitution of India. Besides, the Act seems to be in conflict with the principle of the freedom of movement under Article 19(i)(d) as well as the right to life as provided for under Article 21 of the Constitution (Lawyers Collective 1998).

No other legislation pertaining to HIV/AIDS exists in India. A bill was introduced in the Rajya Sabha on 18 August 1989 which envisaged sweeping powers to the government and health authorities and was, therefore, considered to be intrusive on the liberty of individuals. Health authorities were sought to be provided with policing powers without any accountability under Chapters II and III of the bill. Moreover, the bill had no provisions for obtaining consent, nor did it provide for maintenance of confidentiality. Controversial issues of isolation, quarantine and incarceration were also incorporated in it. Due to the resentment expressed at various forums, and mounting criticism against it, the bill was allowed to lapse. It was considered a classic example of a medical problem being used to further a puritanical, moralistic anti-people agenda, devoid of commonsense and compassion (Goutam 1989). But even after a decade of dropping the move, no further steps have been taken to bring in a more acceptable legislation, despite the numerous handicaps being faced by HIV+ people.

Blood and Blood Products

Different countries have adopted different approaches pertaining to providing compensation to individuals who contract HIV through transfusion of blood or blood products. A French national during the course of a tonsilectomy operation on 29-10-1985 was given three packs of plasma and one ampoule PPSB (a blood product containing coagulation factors). The blood test revealed anomalies and in the year 1987, infectious mononucleosis was diagnosed. Later, in December 1988 and January 1989, tests for HIV indicated positive results. In this case, referred to as FE vs. France, the European Court of Human Rights (ECHR) considered that FE had suffered a loss of opportunities and undeniable pecuniary damages, and awarded him FrF 1,000,000 (ECHR 1998).

In Israel, the government has awarded compensation though it is not liable under Israeli law (Segal 1993). In the United Kingdom, hundreds of haemophilic litigants who contracted HIV through American Factor VII blood products from commercial sources have been awarded compensation. In Canada, even insurance companies have agreed to make substantial payments to their clients (Marshall 1994).

HIV+ people have successfully contested claims against the supply of tainted blood in other European countries such as Italy and the Netherlands, particularly in member countries of the European Community. Of the Asian countries, Japan, among others, has taken a step towards recognising its responsibility for the spread of HIV through blood transfusion (Xinhua 1995).

In Germany, about 60 per cent of over 2,300 HIV+ haemophiliacs contracted HIV between 1983 and 1987 due to the negligence of blood supply companies. The insurance industry did not insist upon proof that a specific blood product had caused HIV. However, payments were confined to loss of earnings and material damages only, not extended to pain and suffering, since German law provides compensation only for proven negligence (World Independent Report 1993).

In order to prevent transmission of HIV through blood transfusion, the Drugs and Cosmetic Act, 1940 in the country was amended by providing that every licensed blood bank shall get a sample of every blood unit tested for freedom from HIV antibodies from such laboratories as may be specified for the purpose by the central government. The date of performing the test is required to be recorded on the label of the container also. This initiative should go a long way in checking HIV infection through blood transfusion in India. But then, the lack of initiative by the concerned authorities, apparently due to financial constraints, has led to judicial intervention. This intervention was occasioned by way of a public interest litigation seeking the protection of the apex court. In fact, it was reported that even after six years of the enforcement of the rules, several hospitals were supplied blood by the Red Cross hospital in Mumbai which was alleged to be contaminated (Mudur 1995a).

The Supreme Court of India has issued elaborate directions by way of guidelines to the government to provide for licensed blood banks in the states and to penalise hospitals and nursing homes in the event of violations of such guidelines. It is heartening to note that in Assam, the State Human Rights Commission took the matter up with the state government in early 1997 to see that the judgement was implemented in right earnest.

Sex, Drugs and HIV

A major route of the spread of HIV in India is heterosexual transmission. The sex trade, although visibly as well as invisibly existent in the country, does not enjoy legal protection for facilitating risk reduction measures. Condom use by sex workers is low. This is also true for couples using contraceptive means for family planning. Prisoners in India cannot be legally provided with contraceptives because homosexual acts are an offence under Section 377 of the Indian Penal Code (IPC). As such, the supply of condoms in jails would amount to aiding and abetting an offence under the existing law. Further, prison manuals provide for segregation of prisoners suffering from contagious diseases. Under such provisions HIV+ prisoners are lodged in separate cells, evoking strong reactions from NGOs (Mudur 1995b). Likewise, there is no provision for the supply of syringes to HIV+ prisoners who are injecting drug users (IDUs). The scenario is compounded by the lack of anti-discriminatory legislation. Even the issue of marriage among HIV+ individuals is engaging judicial scrutiny and regulations governing the insurance industry are yet to be formulated. Legislation needs to address issues of decriminalisation of brothels, drug abuse and therapeutic use of drugs, apart from formulating information and education laws. Such measures would go a long way in adopting a holistic approach to the entire gamut of issues. Such an initiative would perhaps help to supplement and complement the socio-medical strategy to counter the HIV epidemic in India.

It may be pertinent to take note of certain provisions of the Indian Penal Code which need reconsideration in the context of HIV/AIDS. For instance, if a person knowingly indulges in an unlawful or negligent act likely to spread the infection, he or she is liable to punishment with imprisonment up to six months or with fine, under Section 269. In case of an aggravated form of an offence indulged in without just cause or excuse, he or she may be sentenced under Section 270 of the IPC for a term extending to two years or fined. Similarly, in the event of the supply of infected blood resulting in HIV infection, an offence is registered under Section 304. Homosexual and 'unnatural' sex also constitute offences under Section 337 of the Code (Rao 1995). Newer and fairer understanding of human sexual behaviour all over the world and the gradual acknowledgement of people who have sexual relationships with people of the same sex as them in India makes a re-examination of the laws necessary.

The Role of the Judiciary

In general, judicial responses to health issues have been very positive. But unlike in other countries, there has not been much litigation concerning HIV/AIDS in India. The lack of specific legislation may be a responsible factor. Another factor deterring people from approaching the courts may be the lengthy nature of legal proceedings. Apart from the public interest litigation pertaining to blood banks and the Goa case (Smt. Lucy D'Souza, etc. vs. State of Goa and Ors. AIR 1990 Bom 355-361) referred to earlier, there are a couple of other important cases, but as stated considering the diverse nature of issues involved, the amount of litigation has been small.

In a landmark judgement delivered in November 1998, the Bombay High Court ordered the payment of compensation to a casual labourer whose services were terminated upon his being detected as being HIV+. This happened to be the first case when an HIV+ person moved the courts in India (*The Indian Express* 1997).

Recently, in Mr X vs. Hospital Y, a case before the Supreme Court, Mr X, an assistant surgeon claimed damages against the hospital on the grounds of his HIV+ status being disclosed to his bride's family, Rejecting his contention that the hospital authorities ought to have maintained confidentiality, the Supreme Court held that 'the proposed marriage carried with it the health risk to an identifiable person who had to be protected from infection'. The ruling held that Mr X would be guilty of spreading a potentially life-threatening infection, which, being an offence, would be punishable with imprisonment up to two years and with fine. The court held that the right to marry cannot be accepted in absolute terms (Mudur 1998).

Presently, two HIV+ individuals 'A' and 'C' have moved the Bombay High Court, urging it to declare that they too like other individuals have the right to marry and live normal lives. In the pending writ, the petitioners have however contended that a person could marry another, given full knowledge of the other's positive status (*The Indian Express* 1999). There are a few other cases pending adjudication in different courts and it is expected that with the increasing awareness of legal rights, HIV+ persons will either come forward themselves or that public-spirited persons will come forward to assert their claims against discrimination, violation of confidentiality and other issues on their behalf.

Non-governmental Organisations

Non-governmental organisations have an important role to play in bringing about legal awareness so that no form of discrimination may be practised against HIV+ persons. In fact, Lawyers Collective, a leading NGO, (Positive Dialogue 2000) has been instrumental in the field of HIV litigation in the country. Apart from taking up the cases of HIV+ individuals in the courts, it has been devoting itself in bringing about awareness, particularly among the legal community. Towards this end, a public interest group of lawyers and law students has been endeavouring in capacity-building of communities to tackle legal and ethical issues, apart from campaigning for an appropriate legal environment for combating the spread of HIV/AIDS. Dhaliwal (1998) has observed that the aim of the organisation has been to minimise the spread of HIV/AIDS. It has also been instrumental in the establishment of Citizens Collective, a regional network of NGOs in north-east India, which also plans to educate activists on HIV-related legal issues, apart from projecting the need of related legislation in the region. At the state level too, a number of NGOs have been addressing legal issues. In fact, AIDS Prevention Society, a leading NGO, established a cell devoted to legal, ethical and human rights, and has taken up a number of issues apart from training legal personnel for providing much-needed relief to affected people in distress in north-east India.

Conclusion

The preceding discussion has brought about the inadequacy of legislation in respect of discrimination against HIV-infected people in India. In a country such as India, where HIV is posing a serious threat, there is still no legislation on AIDS. Such a law should be framed in a manner capable of ensuring full community participation and integration of people by securing their cooperation and trust. The objective of the law should be welfare-oriented so as to minimise the risk of HIV infection. It has to succeed in creating a positive atmosphere for the modification of risk behaviour and address issues of infected people at the workplace and in prisons, criminal sanctions, family law, public health, information and education, and the like. Only then would such a law be able to serve the social purpose through functional ability.

References/Further Reading

Dhaliwal, M., 1998. 'Combination Drug Therapy: Inaccessibility in the Indian Context'. 12th World AIDS Conference, Geneva.

ECHR, 1998. European Court Human Rights, Strasbourg, Press release, 2 September–30 October.

Goutam, S., 1989. The AIDS Prevention Bill: Protection or Prosecution. The Lawyers Collective.

Grover, A., 1993. 'HIV/AIDS Related Laws in India', in Robert A. Glick (ed.), *Law, Ethics and HIV: Proceedings of the UNDP Inter-Country Consultation.*

Lawyers Collective, 1998. HIV/AIDS: The Law and Ethics Background Paper, vols I and II.

Marshall, J., 1994. *Law Review*, 465: 481–87.

Mallikarjun, S.M., 1998. 'Combating Discrimination Faced by HIV Infected at the Workplace'. 12th World AIDS Conference, Geneva.

Mudur, G., 1998. 'Indian Supreme Court Rules that Positive People Inform Spouses'. *British Medical Journal,* 317.

Mudur, M., 1995a. 'India Hit by Contaminated Blood Scandal'. *British Medical Journal.*

———, 1995b. 'India: Campaigners Urge Check on Spread of HIV', *British Medical Journal.*

NACO, 2000. *Combating HIV/AIDS in India.* Ministry of Health and Family Welfare, Government of India, p. 4.

Positive Dialogue, No. 4, 2000.

Rao, M.N., 1995. 'HIV/AIDS: Socio-Legal Aspects'. Souvenir, Indian Law Institute, pp. 48–50.

Report on Discrimination against People with AIDS, 1983–87. New York: New York City Commissioner of Human Rights, 1987, updated 1988–89.

Segal, J., 1993. 'Health, AIDS, Government, Compensation'. *Jerusalem Post.*

The Indian Express, 4 April 1997. 'Bombay High Court asks Public Sector Industries to Compensate AIDS Patient'.

————, 19 April 1999. 'HIV+ Pair Moves Bombay High Court'.

UNAIDS/WHO, 1998. 'Report on the Global HIV/AIDS Epidemic'. June 1998, pp. 6–8.

Watchers, H., 1995. *HIV Law, Ethics and Human Rights,* ed. D.C. Jayasuria. New Delhi: UNDP.

World Independent Report, 13 November 1993.

Xinhua News Agency, 3 October 1995.

10

The HIV/AIDS Epidemic in India: Looking Ahead

Indrani Gupta and *Samiran Panda*

Introduction

There has been a lot of concern in the recent past around whether or not developing countries such as India are overspending on HIV/AIDS to the detriment of other, more common, public health issues. This issue is closely related to the magnitude of the epidemic. The recent debate around figures between the National AIDS Control Organisation (NACO) and UNAIDS where India maintained that the over 300,000 AIDS-related deaths reported by UNAIDS was an unsubstantiated figure, indicates that it is important for planners to know the extent and the spread of the epidemic, especially if planning involves scarce resources with high opportunity costs (Inter Press Service 2000).

It is also argued that while it is now fashionable to maintain that the epidemic is a development problem, the planning of control and prevention as well as the process of implementation in India do not somehow translate this belief into action (Gupta 2000).

It is important to realise that social and economic factors are not only determinants of HIV/AIDS, they are also important in the speed with which the virus spreads. In addition, these factors determine who would be the most affected by the epidemic. Thus, it is not sufficient to only pay mere lip service to its developmental angle, but also to think of serious way in which the development planning processes might incorporate HIV/AIDS in their agenda, else there is every danger that the epidemic will undermine development itself. Despite several years of control and prevention measures, with significant funding from donors as well as the government, India continues to see a spread of the virus, beyond high-risk groups. How then should one amend the planning process or incorporate the epidemic in the main business of development planning? This chapter discusses some critical issues that need urgent focus if India wants to make a dent in the spread of the epidemic.

The Magnitude of the Epidemic: Should it be given Priority?

In India, where planning is an integral part of the development process, the national government has to play a key role in setting up a proper surveillance system. It has been argued that the HIV/AIDS epidemic in India comprises several small foci of intense epidemics within the country (Nath and Chowdhury 1998). This heterogeneity needs to be taken into account while formulating a national surveillance plan, otherwise the resultant actions at the peripheral levels will either not be focused enough for an area with intense epidemic, or not be relevant in areas of very low prevalence. A better surveillance approach would be to combine sentinel surveillance with behavioural monitoring; while HIV sentinel surveillance systems should be in place generally, behavioural surveillance will be essential in areas that are less affected with HIV, to indicate the vulnerabilities in different subgroups.

An attempt was made in the early 1990s to estimate the magnitude of the epidemic in four different parts of India (the estimate of HIV-infected people ranged from 0.44 to 0.61 million) for groups defined in terms of risk behaviour—high, medium and low (Singh 1993). Sentinel data on pregnant women, out-patient department (OPD) patients and blood donors was used to estimate the size of the low-risk group. For the medium-risk group, HIV sentinel surveillance data from STD clinics was used. Sero-surveillance data was used to estimate the size of the infected in the high-risk group, which comprised female sex workers, injecting drug users (IDUs) and recipients of blood products. NACO estimates that 3.86 million individuals in India are infected with HIV (NACO 2000).

While this kind of effort is very important, one must realise the. problems inherent in such estimation procedures. AIDS surveillance data is often imcomplete in that it does not reflect the actual number of cases, due to inefficient reporting. Moreover, HIV prevalence data has an urban bias, due to the fact that the surveillance sites are mostly located in urban areas, and there seems to be an implicit assumption that high-risk behaviour is mostly confined to these areas. A third issue is the absence of data on the changing incidence patterns in different population groups, due to the lack of prospective cohort studies. Incidence data is key to proper planning and allocation of resources. Finally, it is difficult to monitor the changing trends in the general population, especially for men (infection among antenatal clinic attendees indicate the extent of the infection among women to a certain extent). Till these problems are sorted out to some extent, estimates and projections in India will continue to generate controversy.

While there is a danger of overemphasising the numbers issue, it is important to understand why magnitudes are important. In countries where resources are scarce in relation to their potential uses, estimating the magnitude of an epidemic is critical for taking decisions on allocation of resources, financial as well as non-financial. Estimation includes both current and future estimates, the latter being important for long-term planning and preparedness for an epidemic. Further, estimation should be as disaggregated as possible for a country which has such a tremendous geographical, cultural and epidemiological variation. While aggregating state data could be meaningful for smaller states, for large states such as Uttar Pradesh, with more than 50 districts, even state aggregates may not be relevant.

A last point concerns the demographic impact of the epidemic; by definition, an epidemic will have serious implications for the morbidity and mortality rates and the economy. There is still very little evidence that HIV/AIDS has a serious impact on death rates in India. This could be partly due to the way death records are maintained in India, partly due to the possibility that a bulk of these deaths are not being recorded, and partly due to the fact that the numbers are not large enough to show up in mortality rates. At the same time, since the epidemic has been around for more than a decade and a half, it has to be true that AIDS deaths are taking place in India, in excess of deaths without the epidemic (Eliot 1998). It might be a good opportunity for the government to re-visit and amend its data collection system, especially the SRS (Sample Registration System), to find ways of improving the data on deaths in India. In addition, other existing national data collection efforts such as the NSS (National Sample Survey) and the Census should also be reviewed in the context of the AIDS epidemic.

Determinants of the Spread of HIV: Do We Know Enough?

It is encouraging to note that discussions around how HIV spreads have now gone beyond a mere discussion of high-risk groups to the factors that make individuals susceptible and vulnerable to infection. What makes some people or some groups more vulnerable than others? A related question is—what are the factors that constrain people's ability to understand messages of prevention and control? Answers to both these questions are critical to effective prevention and control measures.

These question are easier to articulate than to answer. There are many and varied factors that go into determining vulnerability. Behaviour is affected by an individual's social, demographic, economic and cultural characteristics; thus age, gender, education, marital status, employment status and living conditions all go to determine susceptibility to infection. The second set of factors comprises those that interact with the micro factors and include all aspects of society—economic, social, cultural, political and legal. These factors are directly linked to policies and programmes, mainly of the national government. For example, micro factors such as employment status and living conditions are directly the result of policies at the macro level. Together, the micro and macro factors determine not only who is most susceptible, but also who is better placed to absorb control and prevention messages.

To take this argument a little further, any marginalised group in society is more vulnerable to the infection—these groups could include women, the unemployed, those living in slums, groups that are declared illegal, etc. At the same time, the fact of their being marginalised in turn affects the availability and accessibility of health care to them. Further, there are macro-administrative and even legal factors that move these individuals away from mainstream life. For example, the treatment meted out to IDUs in hospitals is different and often discriminatory from that given to other individuals (Panda et al. 1998). Similarly, the current laws on sexual issues and obscenity that force men who have sex with men (MSM) underground, make it difficult to reach them for any kind of intervention, thereby increasing their susceptibility to infection (Bandyopadhyay 1998).

NACO mentions labour migration, labour mobility, low literacy and gender disparity as some of the key vulnerability issues in India (NACO 1998–99). At the same time, rural–urban migration creates many distinct vulnerable groups such as slum dwellers, street children and beggars, who are at greater risk. Similarly, adolsecents—girls and boys—women dependent on others and working women are also at risk due to their inability to protect themselves. It is important, therefore, to understand the processes that create vulnerable groups and the factors that continue the vulnerable status of such people and groups. More studies are difinitely needed, especially to understand why prevention measures are not making much of an impact on the vulnerability status of individuals.

A good example is the Sonagachi project in West Bengal. Attempts to bring in change in risk practices with regard to the HIV epidemic through environmental intervention have been the key factor in the Kolkata-based Sonagachi project; this intervention has enabled sex workers to maintain safer sex practices and has kept the HIV and STD prevalence in this group at its present low. Some of these environmental changes came about as a response to the felt needs of the population at risk; an important feature of this process has been the willingness and ability of the project to revise interventions in view of the changing felt needs arising out of the changing environment in the red-light districts. For example, inclusion of sex workers in planning and implementation, constant negotiation and adjustment of the relationship of sex workers with the power brokers in a brothel setting (pimps, madams and the police), and responding to the larger needs of the sex workers in the areas of literacy, education of children, credit facilities, etc., are some of the key elements that went into the creation of an enabling environment in Sonagachi.

Socio-economic Impact: Inadequate Emphasis

This is one area which has been somewhat neglected both in discussions and debates as well as in financial strategies to cope with the epidemic. The impact of the epidemic can be felt broadly at four levels: at the macro or the economy level, at the level of sectors—industry, health, government, etc., on the community, and on individuals and their families. The determinants of impact are, therefore, different at each of these four levels. However, it can be safely assumed that the impact felt at the individual/household level would to a large extent determine the impact at the other levels, and, to that extent, the most immediate concern in impact alleviation interventions must start with the affected individuals and their families.

As mentioned in the previous section, micro and macro factors determine the extent of the impact in any setting. But one important aspect that stands out is poverty—poverty status also determines who gets infected, it impacts more on who is able to cope the best in these circumstances. While poverty status may change over time, at a given point of time—when the person acquires the infection—it is part of her/his personal circumstances. Poverty not only gives rise to economic hardships but also determines a wide range of non-economic aspects, such as, health seeking behaviour, exercise of legal rights and extent of discrimination. Since poverty is one factor that is a given at the time of acquiring the infection, it would be essential to know how it influences the impact of HIV on an individual/household within the sociocultural context.

Care and management of people living with HIV and AIDS (PLWHA) is often narrowed down to only therapeutic management of the disease. It is also seen as an area where resources get drained without any visible returns for the society. Both these myths need to be exploded for effective prevention and control, as well as for tackling the impact of the epidemic in India. Experiences from other developing countries have shown that effective care and management can help the PLWHA to lead productive lives in the community. Moreover, management and care should include issues beyond just therapeutic aspects and focus also on improvement in the quality of life. Financial and other needs of people infected with HIV, the need for information for prevention of further spread of HIV to spouses, care of children in families having members infected with HIV and allowing human dignity to those affected, are some of the issues related to this broader understanding of HIV/AIDS care and management.

At the sectoral level, there is very little that is known for India; for instance, we do not yet know which industry is going to be most affected and how much. What would be the impact on agriculture? What is going to be the impact on the health sector and on the government? These issues need attention both for advocacy purposes and for purposes of policy.

Prevention, Control, Care and Support in India: Context and Limitations

The immediacy of the HIV/AIDS problem prompted a reaction in India which largely mirrored the practices followed by other countries in the prevention and control of HIV/AIDS. The National AIDS Control Organisation responded by putting in place a package comprising surveillance, programme management, information, education and communication (IEC), blood safety, condom promotion, control of STDs, and clinical management. However, these components were set in place without a proper understanding of the need to affect changes in both the immediate environment and the structure in which individuals were operating. For example, it has been argued that the central and state governments have been handicapped by several factors, the most important being the existing public health problems (Dasgupta et al. 1994). The health care delivery system is an area of critical importance, since much of the prevention and control mechanisms take place via this system. Similarly, it is important to understand why certain groups are unable to derive benefit from the IEC materials; the immediate environment differs across groups, making a uniform package of IEC material ineffective in certain cultural or social contexts. This limitation has been recognised by NACO and an ongoing effort is being made to revise the existing IEC materials, based on social and ethnographic research (NACO 1997–98).

On the other hand, NGOs, who are much closer to the grassroots realities, have a greater understanding of the immediate needs of the community and the existing environment. NGOs have often recognised the needs of susceptible groups, which were often over-looked by mainstream interventions. For example, interventions with street children (Karmakar et al. 1998), widows (Devi 1998), shipyard workers (Vaishnav 1998) and the fisherfolk community (Bandyopadhyay and Barman 1998) demonstrate the ability of NGOs to reach out to populations that are hard to access.

There are limitations inherent in the very way the NGOs operate. One important area of concern in NGO interventions arises from the fact that there is inadequate and imperfect understanding of the critical minimum coverage that is required to effectively reduce the incidence of HIV and STDs within the population at risk. Other issues such as inadequate pooling and sharing of experiences as well as resources, lack of research, lack of moni-toring and evaluation, as well as an imperfect understanding of the larger environment, which includes the mode of governance in the country in which they have to operate, have often resulted in well-intentioned interventions not achieving the desired results.

In both government and non-government approaches, one factor has been an unwillingness and/or an inability to understand that even the best designed interventions ultimately would not achieve the desired results, unless the system in which these oper-ate is altered in significant ways. Thus, for example, health inter-ventions that operate through the existing inefficient health care delivery system will have limited impact unless one changes the critical bottlenecks that act as impediments (Dasgupta et al. 1994).

Although the HIV epidemic has already been in the country for more than a decade and a half, adequate and proper government response in care and management is yet to be seen from the cen-tre as well as the states in India. Cases of isolation of and dis-crimination against PLWHA do still happen at government as well as private hospitals (Gupta 1997).

Discrimination against people infected with HIV at the workplace is another important area that needs to be addressed as a part of an effective care and management plan. An experimental intervention plan in this regard at 15 establishments in the city of

Bangalore has been able to tackle peer rejection and management hostility. All the establishments visited for this purpose by a team of doctors, psychologists and industrialists accommodated their HIV+ employees except in one instance where the positive person got a placement at a different establishment (Mallikarjun 1998).

The involvement of NGOs and community-based organisations (CBOs) in care and support of people infected with HIV has also been sparse in India. However, the encouraging model of the 'continuum of care' project developed in the north-eastern state of Manipur could serve as a guiding matrix for developing collaboration between the government, NGOs, CBOs and the community in other parts of the country, so that the care needs of people infected with HIV could be responded to at all levels (Singh 1998).

However, it must be recognised that no national government can fully sponsor a care and support programme on its own, and it is not surprising that this component has not received adequate attention in India. Of course, the government can help by either lending direct support and/or creating an enabling environment for other organisations as well as for the affected individuals and their families to initiate and carry on care and support activities.

Interventions: Formulation and Evaluation

In the case of the National AIDS Control Programme in India, the initial stages saw a top-down approach, with very little emphasis on partnerships. While this approach in combination with a vertical programme implied that HIV/AIDS was finally on the national agenda, the limitations of the approach were soon visible. The formation at the state level of State AIDS Control Society in Tamil Nadu, in contrast to the earlier AIDS Control Cell, is an active attempt to help not only easier disbursement of funds, but also smoother cooperation between the society and its partners—NGOs, CBOs and even other parts of the government sector. It is hoped that more states will benefit from this way of functioning. It is also necessary to intergrate the AIDS programme with other government programmes, such as the Reproductive and Child Health Programme (RCH) or the TB programme, for more cost-effective use of resources.

There are other instances of NACO actively and successfully cooperating with donors and NGOs: in Tamil Nadu, Voluntary

Health Services—a well-known NGO—together with the State AIDS Control Society and USAID, undertook intensive intervention programmes which were executed through NGOs, the private sector and the government of Tamil Nadu, followed by behaviour sentinel surveillance (APAC-VHS 1999). Other examples of cases where the most affected or vulnerable populations have been partners in the process include the widely acclaimed Sonagachi intervention project (where commercial sex workers were active partners in interventions) and lesser known cases such as the Harm Reduction Programme in Kolkata (West Bengal Sexual Health Project 2000) and the Home-based Care Project by ex-IDUs in Manipur (Sharma et al. 1997), where current and ex-IDUs were active partners in interventions.

The issue of productive partnerships brings up another important point that needs to be emphasised here—the ability to identify why a certain intervention was more effective than another, or why a certain intervention did not achieve the desired objective. For example, it has been learnt from HIV prevention work among IDUs in Manipur that outreach to IDUs will first require conducting outreach to the non-drug using community. Given the nature of the problems (marginalisation and discrimination, lack of services in general) it is vital to accomplish this as a first step in facilitating outreach to IDUs (Hangzo et al. 1997). The effectiveness of an intervention is critically related to the issue of forming effective and important primary as well as secondary partnerships; all those directly and indirectly affected by an intervention in whatever capacity need to be taken into confidence at the planning stage, even if the actual implementation of the intervention does not involve all of them.

There are now well established guidelines on how to evaluate outcomes (Coyle et al. 1991, Holtgrave 1998). Essentially, the three important questions that need to be looked into are—What interventions are actually delivered? Do the interventions actually make a difference? What interventions or variations of interventions work better? Currently, there is very little information in India on the last two questions. While formative evaluations undertaken before an intervention is formulated can inform decision-making, these are essentially small-scale efforts. To quantify the interventions that are actually delivered, one needs process evaluation, and to ultimately answer the question of whether or not the interventions make a difference and what works better, one needs outcome evaluations. The requirements for outcome evaluation in terms of information and data are quite daunting, especially the ones involving randomised experiments; however, there is no other scientific way to understand which of the evaluations work better, and though non-experimental or quasi-experimental methods have their limitations, these can often yield useful results and guide interventions.

One of the main issues in such evaluations lies in defining clearly and correctly the programme objectives and selecting precise outcome measures. While evaluating AIDS prevention programmes, it seems intuitively reasonable that prevention of additional infections should be the primary outcome measure. However, infections prevented can often not be directly observed; in such cases behavioural outcomes that can be assumed to lead to lower incidence of infection can be used as surrogate outcome variables. It is, of course, always possible to ultimately quantify, based on different assumptions of transmission rates and incidence, how many infections will be averted, given that behaviour has changed in a certain fashion. The objective of an intervention could also be intervening outcomes such as the number of pregnant women tested, the number of syringes circulated, the number of individuals counselled, etc. However, while these outcomes can be measured, ultimately the effectiveness of all these prevention strategies should be measured in the number of infections averted.

In India, implementors and funders often undertake ex-post evaluations, without realising that proper evaluations need parameter values before the interventions are in place. Benchmark surveys of important indicators are critical for proper evaluation. NGOs often undertake small-scale interventions, without reviewing whether the need still exists, whether it can be replicated and whether they can go to scale with their interventions. Where they have some semblance of an evaluation process, there is still a need to reveiw and update the list of indicators from time to time, to evaluate the process (rather than only the outcome) and to list the constraints in implementation. Thus, evaluation of interventions is a weak area for both government as well as non-governmental organisations. This is also an area where partnerships are important, where both public and private organisations need to bring in individuals or agencies that have the requisite expertise, early in the planning process. Even the state AIDS control programmes need evaluation before the next round of investments are made. This is a very important weakness in the current set-up, and it contribute towards the ineffective use of scarce resources.

Resource Availability and Financial Sustainability

Ideally, all interventions, including those for HIV/AIDS, should be selected on the basis of cost-effectiveness in terms of resources, and should yield maximum benefits at least costs. In developing countries, where resources are scarce for all sectors, but especially for social sectors, carefully thought-out and financially cost-effective interventions are the only ones that can be justified. While the government is the obvious entity that comes to mind, it must be realised that all investment must be cost-effective irrespective of which sector they emanate from. After all, resources have alternative uses, and the government, donors as well as NGOs must undertake to the extent possible some analyses of cost-effectiveness.

However, cost-effectiveness analysis is not easy and requires that careful attention be paid to less obvious aspects such as indirect benefits to others besides those directly affected, indirect benefits in some other ways to the same individuals, and a societal perspective rather than a health provider perspective (World Bank 1997a). Another principle that should guide interventions and improve overall cost-effectiveness is the avoidance of the 'crowding out' effect—there should be an overall net gain, rather than replacement, in efforts to control and prevent HIV/AIDS and alleviate its impact. Finally, it has been recognised by donors such as the World Bank that involving other actors besides just the government can improve cost-effectiveness, since each agent or sector will have its own comparative advantage (ibid.). The same is true of communities or NGOs—they need to build partnerships with the government and other authorities, in the areas where they lack skills, to save on scarce resources.

Allocation of resources should be decided not only on cost-effectiveness analysis but also on priorities—within the health sector as well as within programmes in the health sector. Priority areas are often discussed in terms of burden of diseases (BOD) and not merely in terms of mortality indicators. The idea is to go beyond mere mortality measures to include the quality of life that is affected when disability or morbidity strikes an individual. The quality-adjusted life years (QALYs) approach focuses on developing methods for measuring individual preferences for time spent in different health states for a particular intervention. The newer concept of disability-adjusted life years (DALYs) has been more widely used in the BOD approach; it is based on an incidence perspective and provides an estimate of the number of years of life lost due to premature death, and the number of years of life lived with a disability arising out of new cases of disease or injury (Murray and Lopez 1994). These two components yield the total DALYs lived due to disease or injury. This methodology, first utilised by the World Bank in collaboration with the WHO has since been used for global comparative assessments (ibid. 1996). The BOD approach is now seen as essential in prioritising and resource allocation in the health sector. Once the priority areas and groups are identified, alternatives should be evaluated on the basis of sound cost-effectiveness studies.

Calculations of DALYs require comprehensive data on duration of life lost to different diseases, the value of life lived at different ages, comparison of the time lived with a disability with the time lost due to mortality, and the time preference (Murray 1994). Based on its calculations of the BOD in India, the World Bank has calculated the trends in DALYs lost due to selected diseases in four states of India and come to the conclusion that communicable diseases still predominate in terms of disease burden, especially in the low age groups. A projection till 2020 based on alternative assumptions indicate that DALYs lost due to HIV infections in India are expected to rise significantly upto the year 2010, and decline thereafter (World Bank 1997b).

The BOD results in conjunction with information on the cost-effectiveness of interventions are now seen as essential in the formulation of rational health policies, both domestic and international. Thus, as in other diseases, the burden of the HIV/AIDS epidemic needs to be calculated in India, which only reinforces the need for sound epidemiological and behavioural data, along with reliable data on mortality, morbidity and disability. Further, any planning on this front must recognise the diversity of the country and attempt to collect this data in as disaggregated a form as possible.

Financial sustainability of overall health programmes as well as of specific interventions brings us to an issue that has been mentioned before: that the HIV/AIDS epidemic cannot be tackled by the government alone and it is critical for other sectors, including individuals and households, to recognise this fact. Pooling resources, financial and otherwise, is going to be necessary, especially if the objective of long-term sustainability of intervention efforts is to be met. While prevention and control efforts have large external benefits, socio-economic impact is one area where the need for innovative approaches is critical; this is because private suffering does not typically have other significant negative externalities which can justify the use of a significant share of public money. It has been suggested that individuals and households, armed with the knowledge of HIV status, can start planning early for the future years, especially keeping in view the progressively increasing need for more resources (Gupta 1998).

There is no easy answer to the question of the availability of resources; each country has to evolve its own process of deciding how much to allocate to HIV/AIDS and under which heads. But since the epidemic is still at a stage where one can hope to avoid a disaster like the ones seen in many African countries, it is critical to act now, and to commit finances, even if these are modest, on a long-term basis. Along with this effort should continue the attempt to tap other sectors, especially those with funds—the industrial and other private sectors. In India, the private sector has only recently begun understanding the problem as evidenced by some important interventions being undertaken by the Confederation of Indian Industries (CII) in some of their firms. A study of industrial workers in Delhi (Singh 1999) indicated substantial high-risk behaviour—visits to sex workers were frequent whereas condom use was low among the respondents and their friends (ibid.). While the study found that AIDS awareness was low among both employers as well as workers, the employers often took a short-sighted view of the problems and thought that productivity in their firms would not be affected by the spread of HIV/AIDS. The CII has for some time now taken note of these indicators of low awareness in industry and has launched intervention programmes for prevention of AIDS at the workplace and in industrial settings. These efforts have been actively supported by NACO. While laudable, these efforts need to be scaled up since most of them are concentrated in a few urban areas in a few states.

Planning for Short- and Long-term Interventions

While the need to respond is immediate and calls for action now rather than later, not all planning around the epidemic çan be short-term. Short-term planning and interventions take as given the constraints imposed by the system or the structure in which the individuals operate. But any sustainable intervention design must recognise that there are structural problems which, if not tackled, will set an upper limit to the effectiveness of interventions. Some examples would include the legal system, the health care delivery system, the administrative and enforcement structure of the country and even the political environment.

In India, all programmes must take into account the fact that it is a democratic country, with rights that all individuals have. Any intervention that tries to be authoritarian will ultimately fail by eliciting public opinion against such measures. The legal system is still weak and slow enough to not protect the rights of citizens. For example, while it is illegal to throw a person who is positive out of a job, the legal system is not prompt to protect those who have been thus discriminated against.

Looking Ahead

The HIV/AIDS epidemic has shown up the inherent limitations of short-term and short-sighted policies that do not take into account systemic problems that need to be corrected. These facets are ultimately linked to the overall development of a region or a country or a state. For example, while it is true that short-term interventions can affect a change in behaviour by sending messages about the risks associated with sharing needles, much less is discussed about why the youth of a particular state or region would resort to such practices in the first place. If large proportions of the most productive age group in a population have no jobs and do not go to educational institutions for various reasons, there can only be cosmetiĉ changes with outreach programmes that do not gainfully engage these youths. While 'AIDS is a development problem' has been repeated often enough, none of the policy documents have given any explicit recognition to the processes associated with the 'development' of states in India, which makes large sections of the population susceptible and vulnerable to infection and impact. A National AIDS Control Policy cannot achieve any long-term goals if help is not sought on other fronts—from other departments and ministries, as well as the private sector and communities.

All aspects of life impinging on human circumstances, behaviour and choice affect vulnerability to HIV/AIDS. A vision of how to deal with the HIV/AIDS epidemic has, therefore, to go beyond just this epidemic and plan on a much broader canvas if the lives of millions in this country are to be saved and improved in any significant way.

References/Further Reading

Bandyopadhyay, A., 1998. 'Existing Laws: Impediment to Intervention and Outreach amongst MSM'. 12th World AIDS Conference, Geneva (Abstract No. 60918).

Bandyopadhyay, T. and **S. Barman,** 1998. 'Sexual Health Management Programme for Fishermen Community in Sundarban, West Bengal, India'. 12th World AIDS Conference, Geneva (Abstract No. 43297).

Coyle, Susan L., Robert F. Borusch and **Charles F. Turner** (eds), 1991. *Evaluating AIDS Prevention Programs.* Washington, D.C.: National AcademyPress.

Dasgupta, P.R., M.K. Jain and **T.J. John,** 1994. 'Government Response to HIV/AIDS in India'. *AIDS,* 8(Suppl. 2): S83–S90.

Devi, E., 1998. 'Prevention of HIV Transmission from Injecting Drug Users to their Wives'. 12th World AIDS Conference, Geneva (Abstract No. 60052).

Eliot, Emanuel, 1998. 'Changes in Mortality in Mumbai: Monitoring Mortality to Analyse the Spread of HIV'. In Peter Godwin (ed.), *The Looming Epidemic: The Impact of HIV/AIDS in India.* Mosaic Books.

Gupta, Indrani, 1997. Socioeconomic Impact of HIV/AIDS on Individuals in India. Report submitted to the Department for International Development, United Kingdom. July 1997.

Gupta, Indrani, 1998. 'Planning for the Socioeconomic Impact of the Epidemic: The Costs of being Ill'. In Peter Godwin (ed.), *The Looming Epidemic: The Impact of HIV/AIDS in India*. Mosaic Books.

————, 2000. 'The HIV/AIDS Epidemic in India: Are We Doing Enough?' *Development Bulletin*, no. 52.

Hangzo, C.Z., A. Chatterjee, S. Sarkar, G.T. Zomi, B.C. Deb and **A.S. Abdul-Quader,** 1997. 'Reaching Out Beyond the Hills: HIV Prevention among Injecting Drug Users in Manipur, India'. *Addiction*, vol. 92, pp. 813–20.

Holtgrave, David R., 1998. *Handbook of Economic Evaluation of HIV Prevention Programs*. New York: Plenum Press.

Inter Service 3 July 2000. 'AIDS Scare Reducing Basic Health Funds'.

Karmakar, T., T. Bandyopadhyay and **A Seal,** 1998. 'Assessment of Sexual Health Status among the Street Children in the City of Calcutta'. 12th World AIDS Conference, Geneva (Abstract No. 43245).

Mallikarjun, S.M., 1998. 'Combating Discrimination Faced by HIV Infected at the Work Place'. 12th World AIDS Conference, Geneva (Abstract No. 44178).

Murray, C.J.L., 1994. 'Quantifying the Burden of Disease: The Technical Basis for Disability-Adjusted Life Years'. In C.J.L. Murray and A.D. Lopez (eds), *Global Comparative Assessments in the Health Sector: Disease Burden, Expenditures and Intervention Packages*. Geneva: World Health Organization.

Murray, C.J.L. and **A.D. Lopez** (eds), 1994. *Global Comparative Assessment in the Health Sector: Disease Burden, Expenditures and Intervention Packages*. Geneva: World Health Organization.

————, 1996. *The Global Burden of Disease*. Cambridge, Mass.: Harvard School of Public Health.

Nath, L.M. and **S. Chowdhury,** 1998. 'Many Small Epidemics: Implications for Planning and Interventions'. 12th World AIDS Conference, Geneva (Abstract No. 60432).

National AIDS Control Organisation (NACO), 1997–98. Country Scenario, Update, Ministry of Health and Family Welfare, Government of India.

————, 1998–99. Country Scenario, Update, Ministry of Health and Family Welfare, Government of India.

————, 2000. Combating HIV/AIDS in India, Ministry of Health and Family Welfare, Government of India, p. 4.

Panda, S., A. Chatterjee, S. Bhattacharjee, B. Roy, M.K. Saha and **S.K. Bhattacharya,** 1998. 'HIV Hepatitis B and Sexual Practices in the Street-recruited Injecting Drug Users in Calcutta: Risk Perception versus Observed Risks'. *International Journal of STD & AIDS*, 9: 214–18.

Sharma, H.U., N.R. Singh, A.A. Singh, H.D. Singh and **S. Panda,** 1997. 'Home-based Care Project by Ex-Injecting Drug Users Following HIV Epidemic in Manipur, India'. 3rd International Conference on Home and Community Care for Persons Living with HIV/AIDS, Amsterdam (Abstract No. P145).

Singh, Padam, 1993. 'Projections on AIDS and HIV'. *CARC Calling*, vol. 6, no. 3.

Singh, R., 1999. *Workers and Labour Rights: A Study of Vulnerability of the Workers in Wazirpur Industrial Area*. Delhi: Mimeo.

Singh, V.N., 1998. 'Care in Resource Limited Settings'. 12th World AIDS Conference, Geneva (Abstract No. 12410).

Vaishnav, N., 1998. 'Awareness among Migrant Workers at Shipyard'. 12th World AIDS Conference, Geneva (Abstract No. 60097).

Voluntary Health Services, 1998. HIV Risk Behaviour Surveillance Survey in Tamil Nadu. Report Third Wave 1998.

West Bengal Sexual Health Project, 2000. Partners, February 1(14).

World Bank, 1997a. *Confronting AIDS: Public Priorities in a Global Epidemic.* Oxford University Press.

———, 1997b. India: New Directions in Health Sector Development at the State Level: An Operational Perspective. Report No. 15753-IN.

About the Editors
and Contributors

Editors

SAMIRAN PANDA is an Associate Consultant at the Center for Harm Reduction, MacFarlane Burnet Center for Medical Research, Australia, and Principal Investigator of the Research on Infection and Immunity: Collaborative Effort (RIICE), Society for Applied Studies, Kolkata (India). He is also the Vice President of the Society for Positive Atmosphere and Related Support to HIV/AIDS (SPARSHA), Kolkata. Dr Panda is the recipient of the best scientist award for communicable and infections disease research of the Indian Council of Medical Research in 1996. He has worked extensively in different parts of India, Nepal and Bangladesh as a consultant of DFID, UNAIDS, UNDCP, FHI, AusAID, Sida, PCI and the Population Council for HIV/AIDS prevention and care in different population groups.

ANINDYA CHATTERJEE is the South Asia Coordinator, UNAIDS, Country and Regional Support Department, Geneva. He has worked with governmental bodies, NGOs, and research and international agencies in many parts of India, Bangladesh, Nepal, Iran, Myanmar, China, Indonesia and Thailand. Dr Chatterjee's areas of expertise include HIV prevention programmes for vulnerable populations; rapid assessments of drug use and HIV situation analyses; monitoring and evaluating HIV prevention and behavioural intervention programmes; treatment of drug use; health policy research; and public health advocacy.

ABU S. ABDUL-QUADER is a behavioural scientist based in Atlanta, USA. With over 15 years of experience in the field of HIV/AIDS, he has conducted intervention research targeting injecting drug users and their sexual partners in the USA and in developing countries. Dr Abdul-Quader was formerly associated with St. Luke's Roosevelt Hospital, New York, and the World Health Organization, Geneva.

Contributors

PETER AGGLETON is Professor and Director of the Thomas Coram Research Unit, Institute of Education, University of London, London.

SHALINI BHARAT is Professor in the Unit for Family Studies, Tata Institute of Social Sciences, Mumbai.

DEBASHIS BOSE is Dermato-venereologist of the Sonagachi STD/HIV Intervention Project, Durbar Mahila Samanwaya Committee, Kolkata.

ASHOKE CHATTERJEE is Distinguished Fellow at the National Institute of Design, Ahmedabad.

SANCHITA CHOWDHURY is Senior Research Officer of the Sonagachi STD/HIV Intervention Project, Durbar Mahila Samanwaya Committee, Kolkata.

SUPARNA GHOSH is Junior Research Officer of the Sonagachi STD/HIV Intervention Project, Durbar Mahila Samanwaya Committee, Kolkata.

INDRANI GUPTA is Reader at the Health Policy Research Centre, Institute of Economic Growth, Delhi.

SMARAJIT JANA is the Chief Advisor of the Sonagachi STD/HIV Intervention Project, Durbar Mahila Samanwaya Committee, Kolkata.

M. SURESH KUMAR is a Psychiatrist at the Institute of Mental Health, Chennai.

KAMALA MUKHERJEE is Field Supervisor of the Sonagachi STD/HIV Intervention Project, Durbar Mahila Samanwaya Committee, Kolkata.

K. PRADEEP is the Strategic Planning Officer of UNAIDS, New Delhi.

SUBHRAM RAJKHOWA is Reader, Department of Law, Gauhati University, Guwahati, Assam.

TARUN K. ROY is Director of the International Institute for Population Studies, Mumbai.

KUSUM SAHGAL is the Principal and Superintendent of Lady Hardinge Medical College, New Delhi.

GEETA SETHI is the Country Programme Advisor of UNAIDS, Bangladesh.

RAVI K. VERMA is Programme Associate in the HORIZONS programme of the Population Council, New Delhi. He was formerly associated with the International Institute for Population Studies, Mumbai.

Index